Canine and Feline Nutrition for Veterinary Nurses

Canine and Feline Nutrition for Veterinary Nurses

Nicola Lakeman

WILEY

This edition first published 2027

Registered Offices
John Wiley & Sons, Inc., 111 River Street, Hoboken, NJ 07030, USA
John Wiley & Sons Ltd, New Era House, 8 Oldlands Way, Bognor Regis, West Sussex, PO22 9NQ, UK

For details of our global editorial offices, customer services, and more information about Wiley products visit us at www.wiley.com.

The manufacturer's authorized representative according to the EU General Product Safety Regulation is Wiley-VCH GmbH, Boschstr. 12, 69469 Weinheim, Germany, e-mail: Product_Safety@wiley.com.

Wiley also publishes its books in a variety of electronic formats and by print-on-demand. Some content that appears in standard print versions of this book may not be available in other formats.

Library of Congress Cataloging-in-Publication Data applied for:

Paperback ISBN: 9781394251667

Cover Design: Wiley
Cover Images: sophiecat/Shutterstock, Alena A/Shutterstock

Set in 10.5/13pt STIXTwoText by Straive, Pondicherry, India

Printed and bound by CPI Group (UK) Ltd, Croydon, CR0 4YY

C9781394251667_250926

Contents

Acknowledgements

These are always difficult to write, as the potential to leave someone out is always there. I would like to thank all of my colleagues, past and present, who have been instrumental in shaping me as a veterinary professional. I would also like to thank all of my family members (especially Gavin and Ellena) who have supported me through the process of writing this text and beyond. Lastly, I would like to thank all at Wiley Publishing for motivating me when I struggled with my writing and for publishing the end product.

Introduction

Canine and feline nutrition is advancing all the time. With our understanding of the interactions between the anatomy and physiology of the gastrointestinal tract, the biome and the pet, altering our understanding of the importance of nutrition. Good nutrition is key to good health and improved clinical outcomes. The requirement for nutritional recommendations is critical to every patient that we see in veterinary practice, whether ill or healthy. Prevention of disease is an important role that nutrition can help with.

Every patient, every animal needs to eat; each one of them needs a nutritional assessment and recommendation. This book provides the underpinning knowledge in order to make that nutritional recommendation in veterinary practice.

CHAPTER 1

Anatomy and Physiology

The digestive system is required to ingest, digest, absorb, metabolise and excrete materials that have been obtained for the required nutrients. The digestive system consists of the following:

Oral cavity (lips, tongue and teeth)
Pharynx
Oesophagus
Stomach
Small intestine (comprising duodenum, jejunum and ileum)
Large intestine (caecum, colon, rectum and anus)
Accessory organs (salivary glands, pancreas, gall bladder [in cats and dogs] and the liver)

Although the gastrointestinal (GI) system doesn't include the biome, it should be noted that the biome itself is the largest element of the digestive process and will be discussed as an integral element of digestion throughout this book (Figure 1.1).

ORAL CAVITY

The oral or buccal cavity contains the teeth, tongue and salivary ducts. The cavity is formed by the incisive bone and maxilla forming the upper jaw, the palatine bone (hard palate) and the mandible forming the lower jaw. The functions of the oral cavity include:

Prehension: The lips and tongue are used to pick up or obtain the food. The use of the lips in this process is essential in rabbits and horses.
Mastication: Chewing is used to break down the food into small boluses before swallowing and mixing with saliva.
Lubrication: The bolus of food is mixed with saliva to make swallowing easier.
Digestion: Amylase is present in the saliva of some breeds of dogs (Pitbulls, Golden Retrievers and Labradors) and not in cats [1]. Digestion of some starches starts in the presence of amylase.

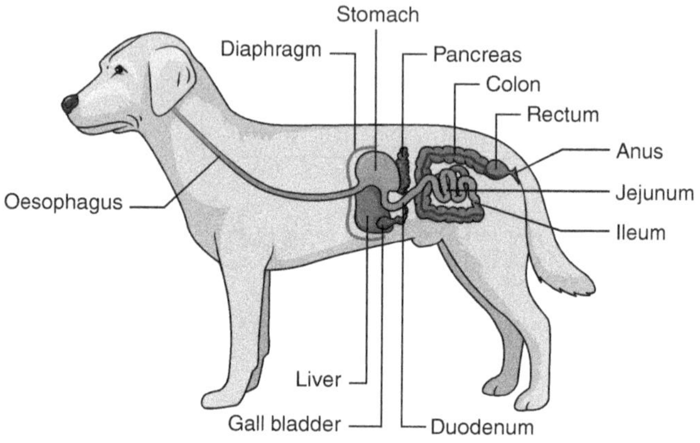

FIGURE 1.1 Diagram of the digestive system.

TEETH

There are two basic types of teeth in mammals, brachyodont and hypsodont. The brachyodont teeth are present in cats and dogs, have a short crown-to-root ratio and have a true root. The hypsodont teeth present in rabbits, horses, guinea pigs and chinchillas have a long crown and a comparatively short root. These teeth are either radicular or aradicular. Horses have radicular teeth, and they eventually form a true root. Rabbits, guinea pigs and chinchillas have aradicular hypsodont teeth [2]; these teeth never form a true root with an apex, and the tooth grows continuously throughout the animal's life. This continuous growth is necessary due to the continual grinding of vegetation during mastication.

Rabbit Formula

$$2 \times \{I2/1 : C0/0 : P3/2 : M3/3\}$$

Dog Formulae

$$\text{Primary teeth} : 2 \times \{Di3/3 : Dc1/1 : Dp3/3\} = 28$$

$$\text{Permanent teeth} : 2 \times \{I3/3 : C1/1 : P4/4 : M2/3\} = 42$$

Cat Formulae

$$\text{Primary teeth} : 2 \times \{Di3/3 : Dc1/1 : Dp3/2\} = 26$$

$$\text{Permanent teeth} : 2 \times \{I3/3 : C1/1 : P3/2 : M1/1\} = 30$$

The action of the teeth is to tear, shred and grind the consumed diet. The tongue helps mix the food with saliva and forms the mixture into a bolus, which the tongue pushes into the pharynx and swallows. Through peristalsis, the bolus moves down the oesophagus into the stomach. The cardiac sphincter marks the entrance to the stomach and relaxes when the pressure from the food bolus builds up behind it.

SALIVARY GLANDS

The salivary glands are situated in pairs around the oral cavity. The saliva, a mixture of 99% water and 1% mucus, enters the cavity via salivary ducts. In omnivores and herbivores, the saliva also contains enzymes. The salivary glands are made up of the zygomatic, sublingual, mandibular and parotid glands. Apart from saliva's function in lubricating the food bolus and enzymatic breakdown (in some species), saliva is also used in thermoregulation. Evaporation of saliva from the tongue (in panting) or hair when applied during grooming helps to cool the animal.

STOMACH

The stomach lies on the left side of the cranial abdomen. The function of the stomach is to act as a reservoir for the food, to break up the food (mechanical digestion) and to begin the process of protein digestion (chemical digestion). The stomach can accommodate the volume of food consumed due to deep longitudinal folds in the stomach wall called rugae. The rugae flatten out as the stomach fills with food. Distension of the stomach stimulates the secretion of gastrin. Gastrin initiates the production of the gastric juices.

The stomach can be divided into three regions: the cardia, fundus and pylorus. Most of the gastric glands are situated within the fundic region (the main body of the stomach). The gastric mucosa (lining of the stomach) contains gastric pits, which consist of three types of cells that secrete gastric juice: goblet, parietal, and chief cells (Table 1.1).

Once food has been broken up and mixed with the gastric juices, the mixture is called chyme. The stomach, via the pyloric sphincter, releases chyme in intervals into the duodenum. This is dependent on the type of food consumed. Foods high in fat will remain in the stomach for longer periods, as digestion takes longer. When the stomach is empty, 'whole organ' contractions occur. This causes the emptying of all swallowed saliva, gastric secretions or refluxed intestinal secretions back into the duodenum. These specific contractions are referred to as housekeeper contractions.

TABLE 1.1 Components and functions of secretions produced by the cells within the gastric mucosa.

Cell type	Gastric juice component	Function
Goblet cell	Mucous	Lubrication; protects the gastric mucosa from autodigestion
Parietal cell	Hydrochloric acid (HCl)	Denatures proteins by creating an acidic environment of pH 1.3–5
Chief cell	Pepsinogen	The HCl converts pepsinogen to pepsin, which hydrolyses proteins into peptides

Rhythmic segmentation occurs in the stomach and through to the large intestines. Rhythmic segmentation is vital in ensuring that chyme is adequately mixed and that absorption of nutrients can occur thoroughly. If this process did not occur, only the nutrients on the outside of the chyme bolus would come in contact with the intestinal lumen and be absorbed.

SMALL INTESTINE

The small intestine is made up of the duodenum, jejunum and ileum. Chyme passes through the small intestine through peristalsis and rhythmic segmentation. The duodenum is in a fixed position due to the short mesentery. The pancreatic duct and common bile duct enter the duodenum. Intrinsic glands (those within the intestinal wall), such as Brunner's glands, secrete digestive enzymes. It is within this initial third of the small intestine where the main portion of mammalian enzymatic digestion occurs. Within the jejunum and ileum, the lumen is where the main nutrient absorption occurs. The intestinal juices are produced by Brunner's glands in the duodenum (these secretions are known as *succus entericus*), and the crypts of Lieberkühn in the jejunum and ileum. The epithelial layer of the small intestine is folded into villi. The function of this folding is to increase the total surface area and increase absorption and digestion. This surface area is further increased by microvilli on the villi, creating a brush border (Figure 1.2).

PANCREAS

The pancreas is a mixed organ, possessing both endocrine and exocrine functions. In the process of digestion, the exocrine portion of the organ is required. The pancreas secretes pancreatic enzymes and bicarbonate, which make up the pancreatic juices (Table 1.2). The juices are secreted into the duodenum via the pancreatic duct.

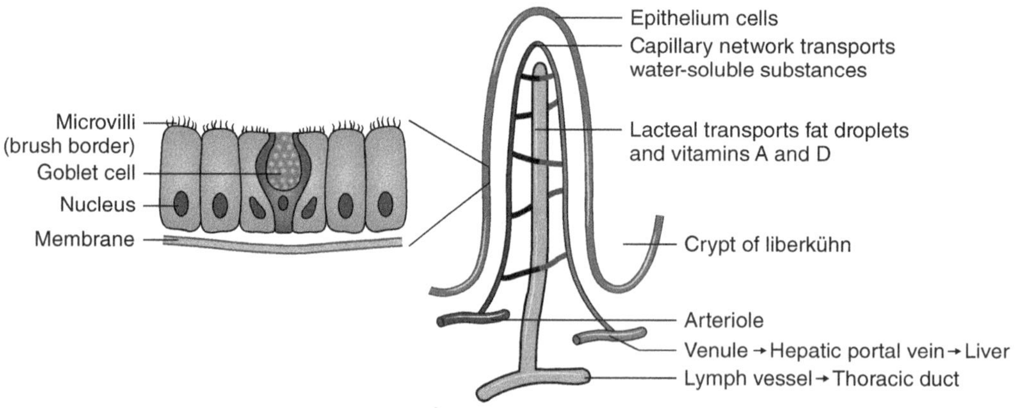

FIGURE 1.2 Diagram of an intestinal villus.

TABLE 1.2 Function of the components of the pancreatic juices.

Component of pancreatic juices	Function
Bicarbonate	Neutralises gastric acid to gain an optimal pH for pancreatic enzymes to work.
Trypsinogen	Converted to trypsin by enterokinase.
Lipase	Activated by bile salts, it converts lipids into glycerol and fatty acids.
Amylase	Breaks down carbohydrates to maltose.
Maltose	Converts maltose to glucose.
Sucrase	Converts sucrose to glucose and fructose.
Lactase	Converts lactose to glucose and galactose.
Enterokinase	Converts trypsinogen to trypsin.
Aminopeptidase	Breaks down peptides to amino acids.

LARGE INTESTINE

The large intestine is made up of the caecum, colon, rectum and anal sphincter (anus). The caecum joins the small intestine at the ileocaecal junction. In carnivores, the caecum serves no significant function, but in hindgut fermenters, the caecum plays a highly significant role. Mammals are unable to digest cellulose; the microflora within the caecum ferment the fibre into short-chain fatty acids (SCFAs) or volatile fatty acids (VFAs), which the animal uses as an energy source.

The ileo-caecal valve divides the small and large intestines. This can be the site of parasitic burdens, especially of tapeworms in equines. The caecum is a vestigial organ in cats, of moderate size in dogs and voluminous and sacculated in horses and rabbits [3]. In rabbits and equines, the caecum acts as a fermentation chamber. Microbial flora break down the cellulose plant cell walls and proteins into VFA. The VFA are absorbed into the circulation through capillaries in the caecal epithelium [3].

In the rabbit, this semi-liquid material passes through to the colon, where the solid, fibrous and indigestible particles are separated through colonic contractions. This material is then passed as hard faeces. The softer, non-fibrous material is passed back into the caecum to undergo further fermentation through retropulsive contractions. This material is excreted as caecotrophs, often at night. These green caecotrophs are rich in protein, vitamins B and K and VFA. The rabbit will usually consume the caecotrophs directly from the anus. Generally, the caecotrophs are covered in a thick mucus. This is to protect it as the caecotroph passes through the stomach into the small intestine, where the nutrients can be absorbed.

The colon is divided into the ascending, transverse and descending colon, and relates to its position within the abdominal cavity. The function of the colon is to absorb water, water-soluble vitamins and electrolytes.

The rectum is classed as the part of the colon running through the pelvic cavity to the anal sphincter. The function of the rectum is to store faeces before defecation. The anal sphincter is made up of two muscular rings, which control the process of defecation. The two sphincters, the internal and external anal sphincters' lumens, are lined with longitudinal folds to allow for the passage of faeces. The internal sphincter is under involuntary control, whereas the external sphincter is controlled voluntarily.

The anal glands (modified sebaceous glands) in cats and dogs are situated between the two anal sphincters. Animals fed on softer, low-fibre diets can have the potential to have difficulties emptying the glands sufficiently enough. Impaction of the glands can result; in these cases, a diet with an increased fibre content is recommended.

THE LIVER

The liver is the largest organ in the body and plays a significant role in the digestion and metabolism of nutrients.

1. Carbohydrate metabolism. The pancreas is responsible for the production of insulin, which allows glucose to enter the cells from the bloodstream. Excess glucose is converted to glycogen by glycogenesis in the liver. The reverse process (glycogenolysis) occurs when the blood glucose levels become low.
2. Protein metabolism. The liver has several roles involving protein metabolism. These include the production of the plasma proteins albumin, fibrinogen, prothrombin and globulin, and the regulation of amino acids in the processes of transamination and deamination.
3. Fat metabolism. The liver converts fatty acids and glycerol into phospholipids and cholesterol for bile salts.
4. Formation of bile. Bile is stored in the gall bladder in some species (e.g. cats and dogs); in herbivores, bile is released into the intestinal tract constantly due to differences in feeding habits.
5. Storage of vitamins, especially the fat-soluble vitamins (A, D, E and K), but also some of the water-soluble vitamins.
6. Storage of iron. Most of this iron is temporary and comes from the breakdown of old erythrocytes and is stored for later use in the manufacture of new erythrocytes in the bone marrow.

Other functions of the liver not related to digestion include the formation of red blood cells in the foetus, storage of blood, breakdown of haemoglobin, hormone production and breakdown, regulation of body temperature and production of heat and the detoxification of harmful substances.

ENDOCRINE SYSTEM

The inclusion of the endocrine system within a nutrition text is mandatory. Interactions of hormones with nutrient intake play a large role in vitamin, mineral and energy utilisation and storage. Understanding the physiology of the endocrine system is required, especially that of the homeostasis of calcium, phosphorous and glucose levels when discussing clinical nutrition.

Calcium and Phosphorus Homeostasis

Secretion of parathyroid hormone (PTH) from the parathyroid glands is dependent on the blood calcium levels (Figure 1.3). When blood calcium levels become low, calcium is resorbed from the bones, and absorption from the intestine is increased. Care should be taken when diagnosing hypocalcaemia, as blood calcium levels can be normal due to calcium resorption from bones occurring, leading to a false positive. Ionised calcium

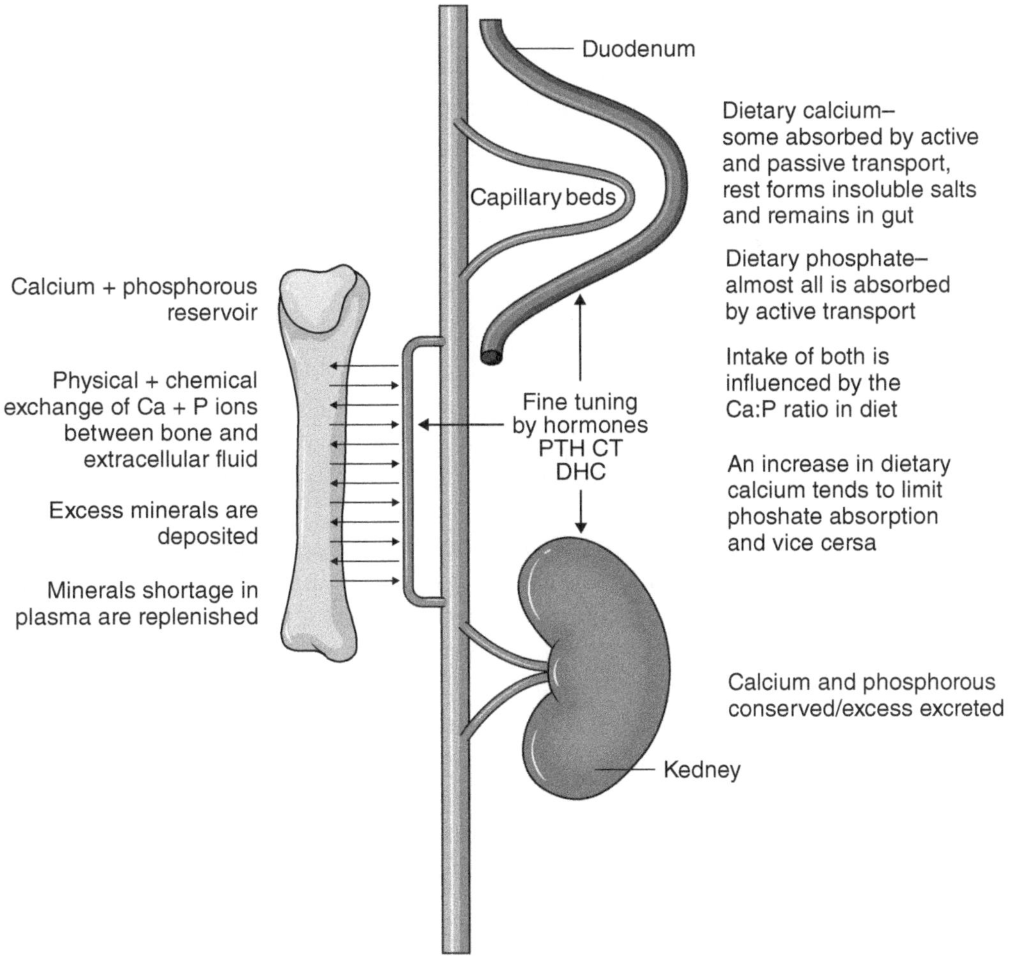

FIGURE 1.3 Calcium and phosphorus homeostasis.

levels should be monitored and requested when submitting blood samples to look at hypocalcaemia. In dogs, a correct calcium level can be calculated to account for this by use of this formula: [4]

$$\text{Correct calcium level(mmol/L)} = ((\text{measured calcium[mmol/L} \times 4) - (\text{albumin[g/dL]/10}) + 3.5) \times 0.25$$

Hyperparathyroidism can occur in three different ways:

1. Primary hyperparathyroidism is caused by direct disease of the parathyroid glands, that is, neoplasia. Clinical signs include bone resorption, bone weakness and pathological fractures.
2. Secondary hyperparathyroidism is seen as a result of chronic renal failure. As the renal function becomes impaired, the ratio of calcium to phosphorus in the blood becomes altered. The consequence of this is an increased secretion of PTH and thus an increased resorption of calcium from bones to maintain homeostasis of calcium levels. With secondary hyperparathyroidism, there is a preferred resorption of calcium from the jawbones (mandible and maxilla), which produces the condition often referred to as 'rubber jaw'.
3. Nutritional hyperparathyroidism results from a nutritional deficiency of calcium in the diet. This is commonly seen in all-meat diets, which also have high phosphorus levels, and in bran diets.

Glucose Homeostasis

The pancreas, a mixed gland, controls the homeostasis of blood glucose levels. The Islets of Langerhans secrete three hormones, which regulate blood glucose levels. The interactions of these hormones aid in obtaining homeostasis throughout the day, as food is consumed and energy is utilised.

1. Insulin (from the beta cells). When the blood glucose levels increase as a response to eating, insulin is released. The action of insulin is to lower the blood glucose levels by enabling cells to uptake the glucose and thus utilise it as a source of energy and by storing excess glucose as glycogen in the liver. This process is known as glycogenesis.
2. Glucagon (from the alpha cells). When blood glucose levels are low, glucagon is released. This hormone stimulates the breakdown of glycogen to glucose (glycogenolysis) in the liver.
3. Somatostatin (from the alpha cells). This hormone is a mild inhibitor of the secretions of insulin and glucagon. This aids in preventing large fluctuations in blood glucose levels.

Diabetes mellitus results from a failure of the animal to produce insulin. This can be a result of many reasons, which are discussed in full in a later section. The role of nutrition is paramount in this condition, as are the routines surrounding feeding (diet, timings and quantities) and daily exercise levels. When trying to stabilise patients suffering from diabetes mellitus, Somogyi over-swings can occur in response to other hormones.

ABSORPTION OF NUTRIENTS

Nutrients are absorbed throughout the intestine and are absorbed in many different means.

- Osmosis or passive transport: This process occurs when a solute moves from an area of high concentration to one of low concentration. This process is not actively used, as once the levels of the nutrient in the bloodstream reach the same concentration as the nutrient in the intestinal lumen, osmosis will stop as an equilibrium state is met.
- Active transport: This process is the main way in which simple carbohydrates, amino acids and peptides are absorbed. Active transport occurs across cell membranes with the use of adenosine triphosphate (ATP). This process is advantageous as it is not dependent on concentration gradients.

The absorption and digestion of fats occur in a more complex manner. Triglycerides present within the diet are emulsified by bile salts within the duodenum. The enzyme lipase is activated by the presence of the bile salts and breaks the triglycerides down into glycerol and fatty acids. Once emulsified and in this state, they are referred to as micelles. The micelles are absorbed into the mucosal cells where triglyceride resynthesis occurs and chylomicron production occurs. These are absorbed through the walls of the intestinal villi into the lacteals. The milky liquid that is formed is chyle and is transported through the lacteals to the cisterna chyli before entering the circulation via the thoracic duct (Figure 1.4).

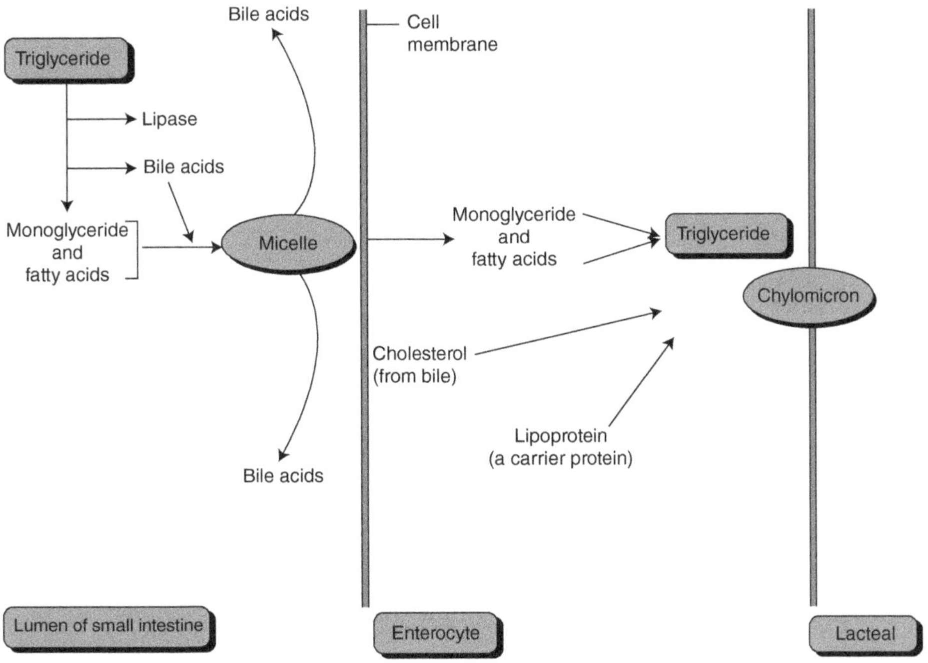

FIGURE 1.4 Diagrammatic representation of fat absorption.

REFERENCES

1. Pajic, P., Pavlidis, K., Dean, K. et al. (2019). Independent amylase gene copy number bursts correlate with dietary preferences in mammals. *eLife* 8: e44628. `https://doi.org/10.7554/eLife.44628`.
2. Gorrel, C. and Derbyshire, S. (2005). *Veterinary Dentistry for Veterinary Nurses*. Elsevier.
3. Aspinall, V. and Cappello, M. (2024). *Introduction to Animal and Veterinary Anatomy and Physiology*, 5e. CABI Publishing.
4. Gough, A. (2004). Calcium disorders of dogs and cats. Part 1: calcium pathophysiology. *UK Vet.* 9 (5): 32–33.

CHAPTER 2

Nutrients

To design or implement a diet for a specific life stage or clinical problem, understanding the nutrient requirements and availability and the consequences of deficiencies or excesses is important. Nutrients are divided into six basic categories:

Water
Proteins
Lipids (fats, oils and waxes)
Carbohydrates
Vitamins
Minerals

WATER

Water is the most vital of all nutrients, and an assessment of hydration levels of all animals should be performed (Box 2.1). When clinically examining an animal, assessing water intake and giving advice to owners on how animals can increase intake is beneficial.

Functions

Water has several important functions within the body. It is required:

- As the solvent for soluble materials (vitamins and hormones) and waste products (urea) is dissolved and transported around the body.
- In chemical reactions that involve hydrolysis, such as the catabolism of other nutrients.

Box 2.1 Factors and parameters that can be used to assess hydration levels

- Tenting of the skin
- Sunken eyes
- Haemoconcentration of blood constituents
- Ability or inability to sweat
- Quantity of urine produced
- Blood pressure
- Capillary refill time (CRT)
- Dryness of the mucus membranes

- In thermoregulation, via the evaporation of water from the tongue (in panting) or skin (in sweating), large amounts of energy are required to evaporate small amounts of water, thus conserving water supplies.
- As a lubricant for body tissues, for example, pleural surfactant and synovial fluids.
- As a major component of blood and lymph, creating a medium for these cells to be circulated in.
- As a major constituent of milk.
- As protection (e.g. embryonic fluids).

Requirements

Body water is lost through urination, defaecation, cutaneous and respiratory routes. Respiratory and cutaneous losses are referred to as inevitable losses, as the animal has no control over them. Water is either derived from metabolic processes or consumed as a liquid or as part of the diet. The daily water requirements of a dog or cat are estimated at 50–60 ml/kg bwt/day and are roughly equivalent to the daily energy requirements (DER) [1]. Consumption of a moist diet will lead to a decrease in the consumption of liquid amounts. Daily water consumption can be greatly increased during lactation and if activity levels increase dramatically. Clinical illness can cause polyuria and thus lead to polydipsia.

Deficiencies

Dehydration in the animal always needs to be corrected before any nutritional requirements are met. Haemoconcentration will greatly alter any blood biochemistries or haematology performed and can be used to assess levels of hydration and any changes over a short period. Table 2.1 shows clinical signs associated with dehydration.

TABLE 2.1 Assessing levels of dehydration in an animal.

Percentage of dehydration	Clinical signs
<5%	No obvious outward signs
	Concentrated urine
5–8%	Slightly prolonged CRT
	Slight tenting of the skin
	Mucus membranes feel tacky
	Third eyelid visible
8–10%	Sunken eyes
	Prolonged CRT
	Obvious skin tenting
10–12%	Oliguria
	Tented skin remains in place
	Clinical shock can be experienced
>12%	Progressive shock
	Death

CRT, capillary refill time.

When calculating daily water requirements, any deficits need to be added to any calculations.

Key Fluid Deficit Formulas:

$$\text{Deficit (ml)} : \text{weight (kilograms)} \times \text{percentage dehydration} \times 10$$
$$\text{Example} : 10\ \text{kg dog}, 10\%\ \text{dehydrated} = 10 \times 10 \times 10 = 1{,}000\ \text{ml.}$$

$$\text{Deficit (litres)} : \text{weight (kilograms)} \times \text{decimal percentage dehydration}$$
$$\text{Example} : 40\ \text{kg dog}, 6\%\ \text{dehydrated} = 40 \times 0.06 = 2.4\text{L.}$$

$$\text{Weight-based loss} : \text{pre-illness weight} - \text{current weight.}$$

Ongoing fluid losses in dogs (vomiting, diarrhoea and polyuria) are calculated by measuring the volume lost over a set period (e.g. weighing soiled pads and measuring urine) and replacing this amount on top of maintenance and deficit needs, typically reassessed every four to six hours.

Key Aspects of Calculating Ongoing Losses.

- **Measurement Methods**:
  - **Vomiting/diarrhoea:** Weigh soiled bedding or pads (1 g = 1 ml). Alternatively, estimate by volume and add to the fluid plan.
  - **Urine output:** Use a urinary catheter to measure or weigh soiled absorbent pads (1 g = 1 ml).

   - **Frequency:** Reassess and adjust fluid rates every four to six hours based on ongoing losses.
- **Formula estimation (if not measured directly)**:

$$4 \times \text{body weight(kg)} \times \text{number of reoccurrences} = \text{volume in ml.}$$

Total Daily Requirement Calculation.

To calculate the total daily requirements, all of the deficits, maintenance and ongoing losses need to be added together.

$$\text{Maintenance (ml)} + \text{Deficit (ml)} + \text{Ongoing losses (ml)} = \text{Daily fluid requirements (ml)}$$

   - Example: 5 kg dog with a 250 ml deficit, 200 ml maintenance and 100 ml ongoing loss = 550 ml total in 24 hours.

Excesses

Excess water is removed via urination. Daily output should be 1–2 ml/kg bwt/h. Water should never be limited unless before anaesthesia or during deprivation testing. Excesses, via over infusion or clinical disease, can lead to pulmonary effusion, oedema or ascites. Polydipsia can result in polyuria and a resulting loss of water-soluble substances, that is, vitamins. For more precise measurements, urinary catheters can be used for urine collection and measurement.

CARBOHYDRATES

Carbohydrates range from simple sugars to dietary fibre. All carbohydrates have the general formula $(CH_2O)_n$ and use hydrolysis when being broken down into mono- or disaccharides. Carbohydrates will tend to have the suffix -ose to indicate a sugar. The suffix -ase tends to indicate the enzyme that is utilised to act on the substrate with the same prefix. Carbohydrates can be subdivided into the following:

- Monosaccharides, simple sugars (e.g. glucose)
- Disaccharides, two sugars bonded together with the loss of one molecule of water, for example,

$$\text{Glucose} + \text{Glucose} = \text{Maltose}$$

$$\text{Glucose} + \text{Fructose} = \text{Sucrose}$$

- Oligosaccharides, three to nine sugar units, for example, raffinose and stachyose.
- Polysaccharides, more than nine sugar units, for example, amylose, amylopectin and glycogen.

Polysaccharides are complex sugars, and the nature of the bonding between the sugar units has a dramatic effect on digestion. Mammalian enzymes such as amylase can only break alpha bonds; only microbial enzymes can break beta bonds. Starches are made up of straight glucose chains of alpha 1.4 bonds (amylose) and alpha 1,6 bonds that form branches. The starch found within plants is called amylopectin, yet within animals, starches are called glycogen. Fibre is an example of a polysaccharide and has an important function in the diet, so much so that it will be discussed separately.

Functions

Carbohydrates are not essential in the diet, as other nutrients (amino acids and glycerol) can be used as precursors of glucose. The presence of carbohydrates within the diet does spare these precursors for their essential functions. The functions of carbohydrates include:

- As an energy source. Energy is provided (adenosine triphosphate; ATP) via glycolysis and the tricarboxylic acid (TCA) cycle (Figure 2.1).
- Can be metabolised for energy to carbon dioxide and water, with the production of heat.
- Once metabolised, can be used as building blocks for other nutrients such as non-essential amino acids, glycoproteins, glycolipids, lactose (important during lactation) and vitamin C.
- Can be stored as glycogen or converted and stored as fat.

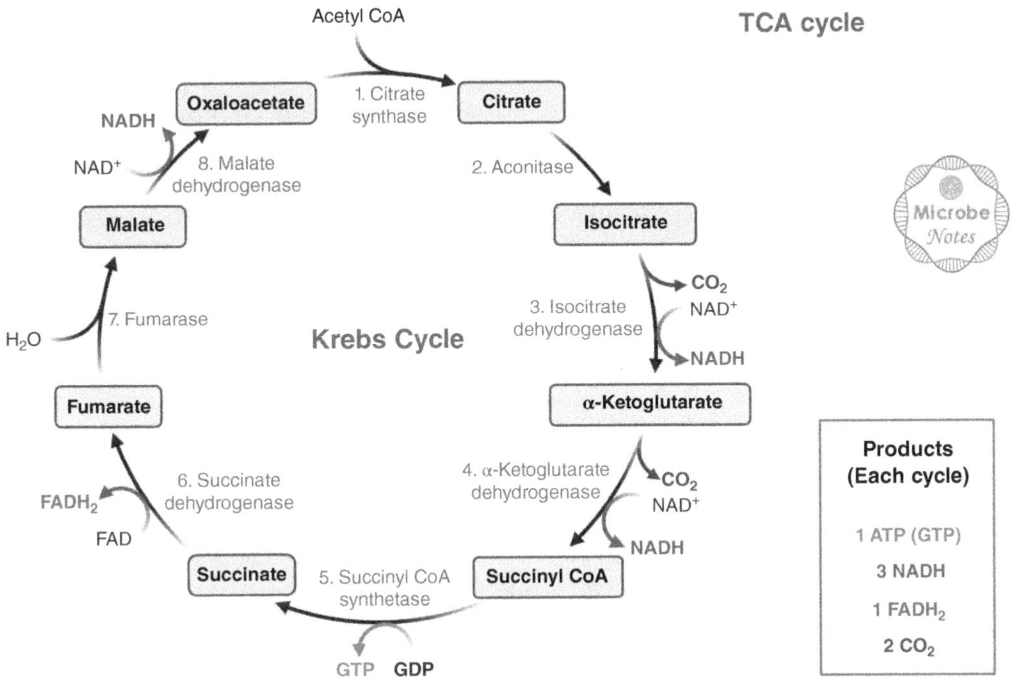

FIGURE 2.1 Biochemical pathways of the TCA cycle. With permission of Microbe Notes.

Requirements

The daily nutritional requirements for carbohydrates are dependent on the energy requirements of the individual. During periods of high energy demands or when new tissue growth is occurring (e.g. growth, gestation or lactation), carbohydrates can be said to be conditionally essential to maintain these metabolic processes.

Deficiencies

Deficiencies in dietary carbohydrates place strain on other metabolic pathways, such as lipids and proteins, to supply glucose precursors. If the provision of adequate glucose is met through these pathways, this can remove these precursors from body protein synthesis requirements. Cats have a unique metabolism and can maintain normal blood glucose levels on a low-carbohydrate, high-protein diet.

Excesses

An excess of dietary carbohydrates can lead to weight gain, as glucose is converted to fat. Because of the previously mentioned metabolic differences between cats and dogs, excessive quantities of carbohydrates in cats can lead to maldigestion (diarrhoea and bloating) and adverse metabolic effects (hyperglycaemia and consequent glucosuria). Persistent hyperglycaemia can lead to glucose intolerance and/or insulin resistance.

FIBRE

Fibre is a complex carbohydrate, but its functions and requirements are different from those of simple sugars and starches. Fibre differs from starch in that fibre resists digestion by mammalian enzymes. Digestion occurs in the colon in dogs and cats and the caecum in horses and rabbits, by microbes. This process, when utilised in rabbits, is regarded as hindgut fermentation. Evolutionary adaptation of the caecum has occurred to accommodate this process. Fibres include cellulose, hemicellulose, pectin, gums and resistant starches. Fibre can be subdivided according to its solubility in water.

Soluble – Pectin, fructans and galactans
Insoluble – cellulose, hemicellulose and lignin

or biologically, according to its utilisation by intestinal bacteria:

Rapidly fermentable – fructans, galactans and guar gum
Moderately fermentable – pectin, beet pulp
Slowly fermentable – cellulose

Functions

Fibre is not classified as a nutrient, but its inclusion within the diet can be highly beneficial for digestive health. Fibre affects the functioning of the gastrointestinal tract by:

- Delaying gastric emptying
- Altering nutrient absorption and metabolism (can be advantageous and disadvantageous)
- Normalising gastrointestinal transit time
- Aiding in the maintenance of the structural integrity of the gastrointestinal mucosa
- Increasing bulk and water in the intestinal contents
- Decreasing overall digestibility of the diet

Requirements

Fibre is not considered an essential component of the diet, and individual requirements will differ depending on life stage and clinical requirements. In healthy animals, a small amount of fibre (less than 5%) [2] that contains both soluble and insoluble fibres is required. Table 2.2 details the effects of dietary fibre on physiological function in the animal.

Deficiencies

Fibre deficiencies are not commonly noted in cats or dogs. However, deficiencies in the hindgut fermenters, rabbits and horses, can be very damaging. Low levels of fibre can result in dental problems and diarrhoea (especially in rabbits). In cats and dogs, dietary fibre is recommended as it produces SCFA/volatile fatty acids (VFA), which the gut microbiota use as an energy source.

TABLE 2.2 Effects of fibre on the physiological functioning of animals.

Physiological function	Soluble/fermentable fibre	Insoluble/non-fermentable fibre
Gastric emptying	Decreased	Some increase
Pancreatic secretion	No effect	No effect
Nutrient absorption	No effect	No effect
Small intestinal transit	Decreased	Increased
Large intestinal transit	Decreased	Increased
Intestinal mucosal mass	Increased	No effect
Microbial growth	Increased	No effect
Toxin binding	No effect	Increased

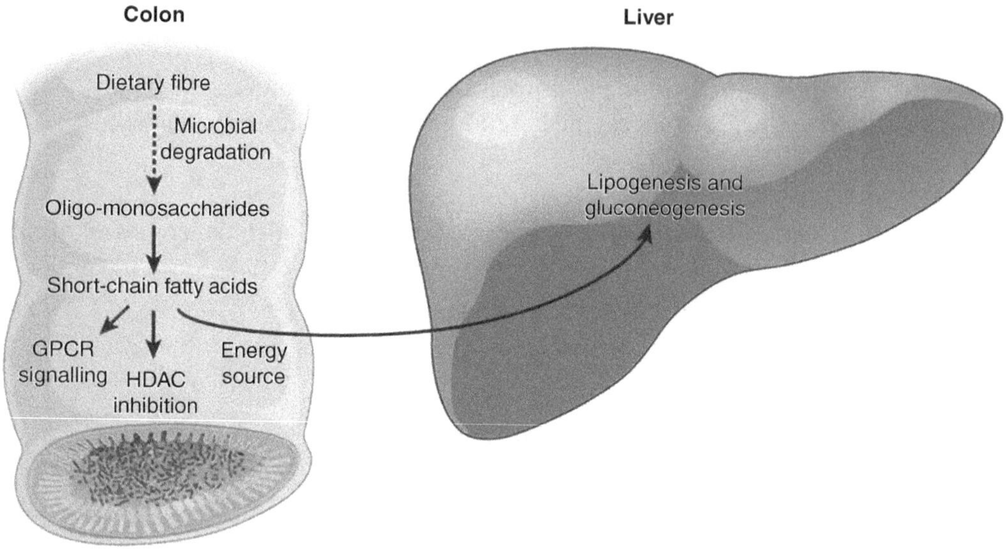

Tremaroli et al. (2012) / Springer Nature / https://www.researchgate.net/figure/Effects-of-colonic-fermentation-of-dietary-fibers-11-Reprinted-by-permission-from_fig3_320674911 / last accessed Aug. 20, 2026.

Short-chain fatty acids are absorbed in the colon, where butyrate provides energy for colonic epithelial cells, and acetate and propionate reach the liver and peripheral organs, where they are substrates for gluconeogenesis and lipogenesis.

Excesses

Excess amounts of fibre can cause the binding of required nutrients, such as minerals. If deficiencies in minerals are identified, consideration should be made of dietary fibre levels.

PROTEINS

Proteins consist of polypeptide chains of amino acids. There are 23 naturally occurring amino acids, which can be bonded into an infinite variety of proteins. All amino acids have the same base groups.

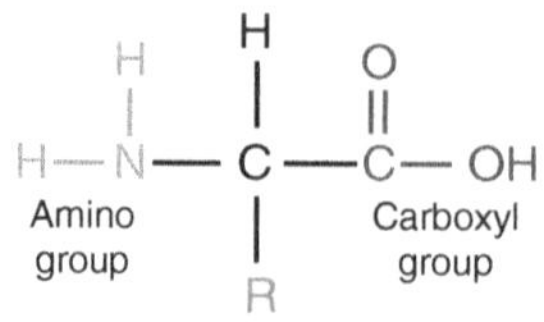

All amino acids contain an amino group, —NH2, and a carboxylic acid group, —COOH. The 'R' is what differs; it can be from a single atom through to complex chains.

Proteins can combine with nonprotein sources (e.g. iron) to form conjugated proteins (e.g. haemoglobin). Amino acids can be divided into two groups: essential and non-essential. Essential amino acids are those that cannot be synthesised within the

TABLE 2.3 Biological values of certain foodstuffs.

Food	Biological value	
	As percentage	As decimal
Egg	100	1
Milk	92	0.92
Meat	78 (variable)	0.78
Soy	74	0.74
Wheat	48 (variable)	0.48

body and must be obtained from the diet. Some amino acids, such as cystine and tyrosine, can be described as conditionally essential. They are only essential when the diet is deficient in methionine and phenylalanine. The ten essential amino acids in the dog are:

Arginine, histidine, isoleucine, leucine, lysine, methionine, phenylalanine, threonine, tryptophan and valine.

The cat requires the same 10 amino acids plus taurine.

The quality or biological value (BV) of proteins is the quantity of that protein (and its composite amino acids) that can be utilised by the animal. The BV can be expressed as a percentage or as a decimal. BV can be applied to all nutrients (carbohydrates and fatty acids) but is primarily used for proteins. A high-quality protein that has a high BV will contain all of the essential amino acids, with high digestibility and bioavailability. Egg has a BV of 100%, cereals a BV of ~40–50% (this value will differ depending on the soil grown in and the type of cereal). Table 2.3 demonstrates some BVs of certain food types.

Commercial food labels are not required to state the BV of the contained proteins, only the percentage of protein as fed or on a dry matter basis (DMB). Confusion can occur when interpreting the quantity of dietary levels of the proteins rather than the quality. Detailed analysis of the BV of the ingredients is also required.

Functions

- Proteins are primarily used as structural components of body organs and tissues, including:
  - Collagen and elastin are present in the soft tissues of the musculoskeletal system
  - The contractile proteins actin and myosin are used in muscle contraction
  - Keratin proteins, within the skin, hair and nails
  - Blood proteins, including haemoglobin, albumin and globulin
- Proteins function as enzymes, hormones and antibodies.
- They are used as an energy source after the process of deamination.
- They are used as the nitrogen source for further production of DNA and other nitrogen-containing substances.

Requirements

The body is in a constant state of regeneration and flux, and the requirement for protein is constant. It can be increased during phases of growth, gestation and lactation, but also when there are inadequate supplies of carbohydrates for energy. Illness and tissue regeneration will also increase requirements; burns and scalds require larger amounts of protein than any other illness. Protein requirements for an adult dog and cat (on a DMB) are 18% and 26%, respectively, and for puppies and kittens, 22% and 30%, based on the Association of American Feed Control Officials (AAFCO) recommendations. This is based on a diet with commonly available protein sources. If the protein fed is of high quality, these values can be decreased, demonstrating the importance of using high-quality proteins in low (quantity) protein diets. The requirements in diets specifically for different therapeutic requirements are discussed in later sections.

Deficiencies

Initial deficiencies in protein can cause the clinical signs of reduced growth rates, poor skin and coat, anaemia, alopecia, reduction in fertility, prolonged healing times, reduction in immunity and a reduction in milk production during lactation. If protein deficiencies continue, a reduction in lean body mass will occur, resulting in muscle atrophy and a reduction in blood levels of albumin and other blood proteins.

Excesses

Protein or amino acid toxicity is not a practical problem in healthy animals due to the deamination process. High protein levels can cause problems in diseased animals, especially those with liver or kidney disease, where the deamination and removal of waste products are impaired. High-protein diets can also prove to be problematic when struvite dissolution is required or when adverse food reactions (AFR) occur within the animal. Additional protein (over and above recommended amounts) in the diet does not have any positive effects. Excessive amounts are converted (deamination) to energy sources. Diets aimed at adult maintenance should not exceed 30% (DMB) in dogs and 45% (DMB) in cats [2].

LIPIDS

Lipids are made of fats (which are solid at room temperature), oils (liquid at room temperature) and waxes. Lipids can be subdivided into single lipids and conjugated lipids. The single lipids include short-, medium- and long-chained fatty acids and esters of fatty acids with glycerol. Of these single lipids, triglycerides are the most commonly found in food. Conjugated lipids and lipids which have combined with other products, for example, phospholipids (used in cell membranes).

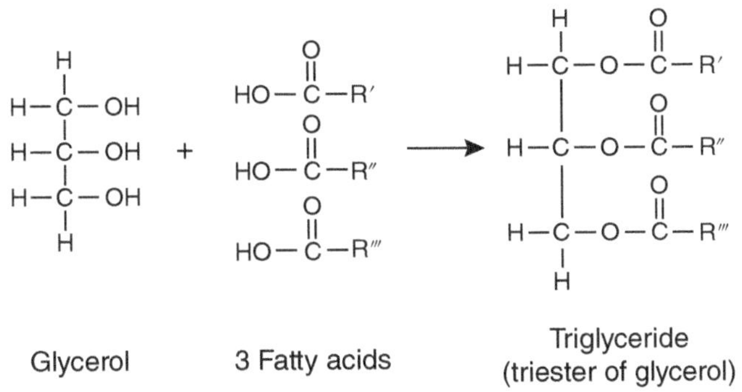

Fatty acids with the first double bond between the third and fourth carbon belong to the *n*-3 group; when the bond is between the sixth and seventh carbon, they belong to the *n*-6 group.

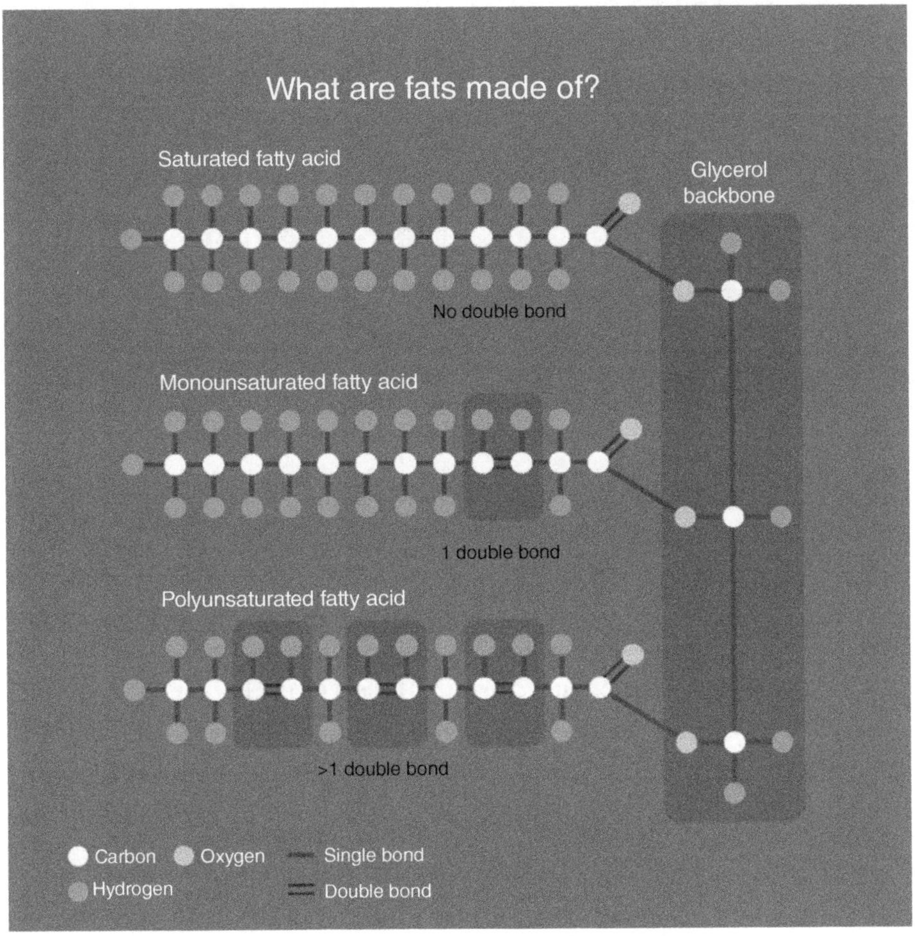

The *n*-3 and *n*-6 fatty acids are the essential fatty acids (EFAs), as animals cannot synthesise these themselves. EFAs in the dog and cat include linolenic (*n*-3) and linoleic acid (*n*-6); arachidonic acid (*n*-6) is also essential in the cat. Adult dogs can synthesise linolenic and arachidonic acid from linolenic acid. Adult cats can synthesise linolenic acid but not arachidonic acid. It was thought that arachidonic acid could only be found in fat sources from other animals, but algae have been shown to have high concentrations. Other important *n*-3 fatty acids include eicosapentaenoic (EPA) and docosahexaenoic (DHA) acids.

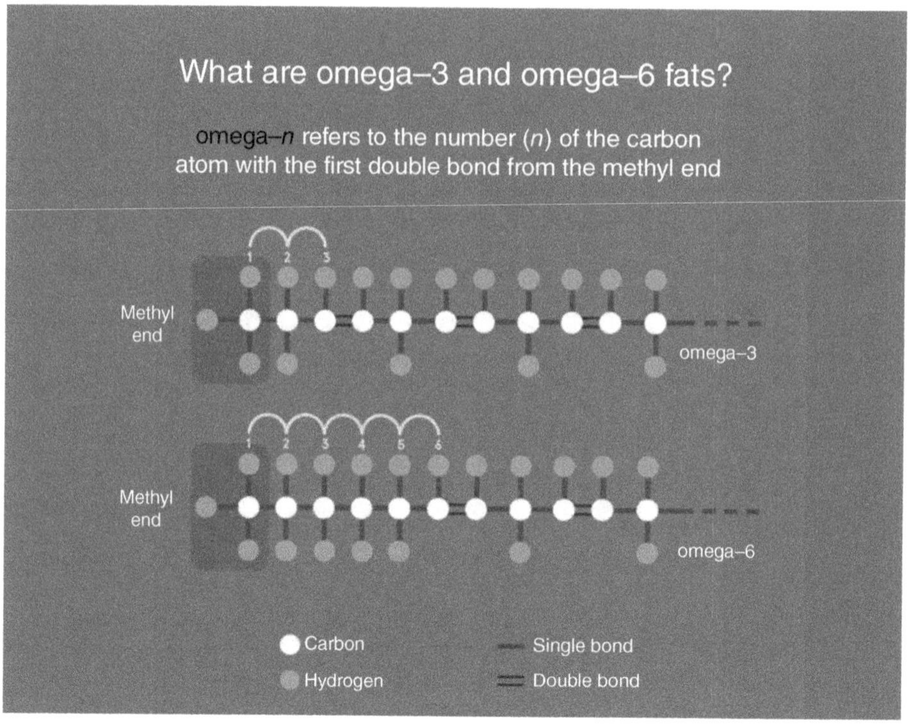

Short-chain	C2	Acetic acid	CH_3**COOH**	*aceto* = vinegar
	C4	Butyric acid or butyrate	$CH_3(CH_2)_2$**COOH**	*butyr* = butter
Medium-chain	C6	Caproic acid	$CH_3(CH_2)_4$**COOH**	*capri* = goat
	C8	Caprylic acid	$CH_3(CH_2)_6$**COOH**	
	C10	Capric acid	$CH_3(CH_2)_8$**COOH**	
	C12	Lauric acid	$CH_3(CH_2)_{10}$**COOH**	*lauri* = laurel
Long-chain	C14	Myristic acid	$CH_3(CH_2)_{12}$**COOH**	*myrist* = anoint, ointment
	C16	Palmitic	$CH_3(CH_2)_{14}$**COOH**	
	C18	Stearic acid	$CH_3(CH_2)_{16}$**COOH**	*stear* = fat, suet
	C20	Arachidic or eicosanoic acid	$CH_3(CH_2)_{18}$**COOH**	*arachis* = a leguminous plant, present in peanut oil
	C22	Behenic or docosanoic acid	$CH_3(CH_2)_{20}$**COOH**	Present peanut and canola oils

Saturated fats

Short-chain	C2	Acetic acid	CH_3**COOH**	*aceto* = vinegar
	C4	Butyric acid or butyrate	$CH_3(CH_2)_2$**COOH**	*butyr* = butter
Medium-chain	C6	Caproic acid	$CH_3(CH_2)_4$**COOH**	*capri* = goat
	C8	Caprylic acid	$CH_3(CH_2)_6$**COOH**	
	C10	Capric acid	$CH_3(CH_2)_8$**COOH**	
	C12	Lauric acid	$CH_3(CH_2)_{10}$**COOH**	*lauri* = laurel
Long-chain	C14	Myristic acid	$CH_3(CH_2)_{12}$**COOH**	*myrist* = anoint, ointment
	C16	Palmitic	$CH_3(CH_2)_{14}$**COOH**	
	C18	Stearic acid	$CH_3(CH_2)_{16}$**COOH**	*stear* = fat, suet
	C20	Arachidic or eicosanoic acid	$CH_3(CH_2)_{18}$**COOH**	*arachis* = a leguminous plant, present in peanut oil
	C22	Behenic or docosanoic acid	$CH_3(CH_2)_{20}$**COOH**	Present peanut and canola oils
Unsaturated fats				

Functions

Lipids have many functions, which include:

- Meeting energy requirements – on a weight basis, dietary fat is approximately 2.25 times more energy-dense than protein and carbohydrates. When stored as adipose tissue, the quantity of energy available per gram is double that of carbohydrates.
- Absorption of the fat-soluble vitamins A, D, E and K.
- Phospholipids are required for structural support (e.g. cell membranes).
- Insulation is especially important in certain mammals in cold climates.
- Hormones, for example aldosterone and prostaglandins.
- Manufacture of eicosanoids.
- Waterproofing of fur and feathers.
- Improving the palatability of foods.

Requirements

The absolute requirement for lipids is an adequate supply of EFA. The use of lipids as an energy supply can be exceptionally beneficial, especially in animals with high energy requirements. Increased fat utilisation occurs during aerobic exercise.

Deficiencies

Deficiencies in lipids can cause a dry coat and scaly skin. A reduction of lipids on the skin can cause a predisposition to pyoderma. Wound healing can also be impaired due to the requirement of phospholipids within cell membranes. If there is a chronic deficiency of lipids, especially of the EFAs, symptoms of alopecia, oedema and moist dermatitis can occur. Severe deficiencies can result in emaciation of the animal.

Excesses

Increased quantities of lipids within the diet directly relate to an increase in the energy density of the diet. Excess fat is stored as adipose in the tissues and around the internal organs. Obesity can arise if excess energy intake and expenditure occur. Excess fats in the diet can predispose the dog to pancreatitis and hyperlipidaemia.

VITAMINS

Vitamins are organic compounds that are essential in small amounts for the normal physiological functioning of the body. Not all vitamins are essential in all species; for example, vitamin C is essential for guinea pigs, but not for cats and dogs. Vitamins can be described as fat-soluble or water-soluble. The fat-soluble vitamins (A, D, E and K) are absorbed from the gastrointestinal tract alongside fats and are stored (with the fat) within the body. Daily intake is not always required because of the quantities sorted and intestinal microbial production (Table 2.4).

The water-soluble vitamins (B complex and C) are absorbed via the gastrointestinal tract but can be lost in the urine. Supplementation of these vitamins may be required when polyuria is present (Table 2.5).

MINERALS

A mineral is the term used to describe all the inorganic substances and elements (including salts) within the body and diet. These substances constitute the ash component of the diet and make up less than 1% of total body weight. Minerals can be divided into three subgroups based on the amounts required by the body.

Macrominerals

Macrominerals are expressed as parts per hundred (pph), with 1 pph = 10 g/kg diet. Their function, sources, deficiencies and excesses are described in Table 2.6.

Microminerals

Microminerals are expressed as parts per million (ppm), with 1 ppm = 1 mg/kg diet. Their functions, sources, deficiencies and excesses are described in Table 2.7.

Trace Elements

These minerals act as catalysts at a cellular level: the amounts required in the diet are not yet known. It is thought that the quantities would be expressed as μg/kg of diet.

TABLE 2.4 The function of fat-soluble vitamins, and the consequences of deficiencies and toxicities.

Vitamin	Function	Source	Deficiencies	Toxicity
Vitamin A (retinol)	Component of the visual pigments in the Eye. Involved in cell Differentiation and Maintenance of cell	Liver, cod liver oil, kidneys and egg yolk	Night blindness infertility, crusting lesions of the nares, seborrhoeic coat conditions, increased susceptibility to microbial infections.	Liver damage, ankylosis of the joints, particularly cervical vertebrae and the long bones of the forelimbs
Vitamin D	Stimulates calcium absorption from the intestine. Participates resorption of calcium from the bones	Can be synthesized from lipid com-pounds in the skin following exposure	Rickets in the young, and osteomalacia in adults	Can result in hypercalcaemia, which if prolonged results in extensive calcification of the soft tissues, lungs, kidneys and stomach. Deforms the teeth and jaw
Vitamin E	Protects cell membranes against oxidative damage	Liver, fats and wheat germ	Pansteatitis (yellow fat disease). Skeletal muscle dystrophy, reproductive failure and impairment of the immune response in dogs	Very unlikely to occur, because relatively high doses are well tolerated
Vitamin K	Regulates the formation of clotting factors (factors VII, IX, X and XII)	Bacterial synthesis in the intestines. Also found in green vegetables	Unlikely to occur Owing to synthesis of the vitamin by intestinal bacteria, unless a vitamin K antagonist has been consumed	Can cause anaemia and other blood abnormalities in young animals.

TABLE 2.5 The function of water-soluble vitamins and consequences of deficiencies and toxicities.

Vitamin	Function	Source	Deficiency	Toxicity
Vitamin B (thiamin)	Involved in carbohydrate metabolism and maintenance of the nervous system	Yeast, fish, egg yolks, cereals and green vegetables	Anorexia and neurological disorders. It can be induced if large amounts of raw fish are fed – it contains the enzyme thiaminase	Thiamin has a low toxicity
Vitamin B_2 (riboflavin)	Essential for cellular growth, carbohydrate, fat and protein metabolism and correct growth	Liver, kidneys, milk, eggs and cereals. Some synthesis in the intestines	Lesions of the eyes, skin disorders and testicular hypoplasia	Not reported
Pantothenic acid	A constituent of coenzyme A, essential for carbohydrate, fat and amino acid metabolism	Liver, kidneys, eggs and wheat germ	Fatty liver, gastrointestinal disturbances, convulsions and depressed growth	Not reported
Niacin (nicotinamide and nicotinic acid)	A component of two coenzymes, which are required for oxidation-reduction necessary for the utilisation of all major nutrients	Meats, liver, fish, rice, potatoes and pulses	Can cause 'black tongue' in cats and dogs	Not considered toxic
Vitamin B_6 (pyridoxine)	Involved in numerous enzyme systems that are associated with nitrogen and amino acid metabolism	Muscle meats, eggs, cereals and vegetables	Anorexia, weight loss and anaemia	Not considered toxic

Biotin B_7	Aids in maintaining the integrity of keratinised structures (hair and nails). Also required for the metabolism of fats and amino acids	Bacterial synthesis within the intestines. Dietary sources can be from liver, kidneys, egg yolk, milk and yeast	Dry, scaly skin, brittle hair, hyperkeratosis, pruritus and skin ulcers. Care should be taken after periods of antimicrobial use or if raw egg whites, which contain avidin, are fed	Not reported
Folic acid	Maturation of red blood cells within the bone marrow. Nucleic acid synthesis and cell replication	Fish, liver, kidneys and yeast are also synthesised within the intestines	Anaemia and leucopenia, but deficiency is unlikely because of intestinal bacterial synthesis	Not reported
Vitamin B_{12} (cyanocobalamin)	Function closely linked to that of folic acid. Also involved in fat and carbohydrate metabolism	Liver, kidneys and heart	Pernicious anaemia and neurological signs	Not reported
Vitamin C (ascorbic acid)	Wound healing, capillary and mucosal integrity	Normally synthesised from glucose. Guinea pigs and humans need to obtain it from the diet (fresh fruit and vegetables)	Scurvy	Not reported

TABLE 2.6 The function and source of macrominerals, and the consequences of deficiencies and excesses.

Macromineral	Function	Source	Deficiency	Toxicity
Calcium (Ca)	Maintaining structural rigidity of bones and teeth, blood clotting, muscle and nerve function and enzyme activation	Milk, eggs and green vegetables	Nutritional secondary hyperparathyroidism. In lactating bitches, hypocalcaemia results in eclampsia. Nervous disturbances	Conditions relating to excessive calcium intake during growth, including hip dysplasia, osteochondrosis and Wobbler syndrome
Chloride (Cl^-)	Maintenance of osmotic pressure, acid–base and water balance. A major component of bile and hydrochloric acid (gastric juices)	Common salt	Inability to maintain water balance, retarded growth, fatigue	Greater than normal fluid intake and consequently polyuria
Magnesium (Mg)	Required for healthy teeth and bones, energy metabolism and enzyme activation	Meat and green vegetables	Muscular weakness	With very high intakes there is an association with an increased incidence of feline lower urinary tract disease (FLUTD)
Phosphorus (P)	Development of teeth and bones, energy utilisation, phospholipids in cell membranes and constituents of nucleic acids	Milk, eggs and green vegetables		If calcium levels are correspondingly low, the ratio of calcium to phosphorus is imbalanced, and hypocalcaemia is induced
Potassium (K)	Nerve and muscle function and energy metabolism are required for acid–base balance and osmoregulation of the body fluids	Meat, fruit and vegetables	Muscular weakness, retarded development, decreased water intake, inability to maintain water balance, dry skin and alopecia	Greater than normal water intake
Sodium (Na)	Muscle and nerve action. Maintenance of osmotic pressure, acid–base and water balance	Common salt, milk, meat, eggs and vegetables	Fatigue, exhaustion, inability to maintain water balance	Greater than normal fluid intake, polydipsia and polyuria can be noted

TABLE 2.7 The function and source of microminerals, and consequences of deficiencies and excesses.

Micromineral	Function	Source	Deficiency	Toxicity
Copper (Cu)	Formation and activity of red blood cells, cofactors in many enzyme systems and normal pigmentation (melanin) of skin and hair	Liver, meat and fish	Anaemia, decreased haemoglobin synthesis. Bone disorders can also occur	Can also cause anaemia. Copper toxicosis can occur because of an inherited defect, resulting in hepatitis and cirrhosis
Iodine (I)	Component of the thyroid hormones, which regulate metabolism	Fish, shellfish	Goitre, hypothyroidism. Clinical signs include skin and hair abnormalities and lethargy. Abnormal calcium metabolism and reproductive failure	Acute effects are similar to those of a deficiency. Toxicity can impair thyroid hormone synthesis and produce toxic goitre
Iron (Fe)	An essential component of haemoglobin and myoglobin, present in many coenzymes involved in cellular respiration	Liver, meat, green vegetables	Anaemia with weakness and fatigue	Anorexia and weight loss in dogs
Manganese (Mn)	Required for carbohydrate and lipid metabolism, growth factor in bone development, enzyme activator and component of connective tissue	Liver, Kidneys	Defective growth and reproduction. Disturbances in metabolism, especially of lipids	Nor reported
Selenium (Se)	An obligatory component of glutathione peroxidase, an antioxidant. Linked with vitamin E and can replace it to some degree	Meat, offal and cereals	Degeneration of skeletal and cardiac muscles in dogs. In other species, reproductive disorders and oedema	Highly toxic in large doses
Zinc (Zn)	Components of enzyme systems, metabolism of proteins and carbohydrates. Essential for maintaining healthy skin and coat	Liver, fish and shellfish	Poor growth, anorexia, testicular atrophy, emaciation and skin lesions. Marginal deficiencies can present as poor skin and coat condition	Relatively non-toxic

Examples of trace elements include chromium, cobalt, fluorine, molybdenum, nickel, silicon, sulphur and vanadium.

ANTIOXIDANTS

The use of antioxidants in the diet is becoming more widely recognised as a positive influence in the health of animals and humans (see Table 2.8). Antioxidants are used to neutralise the ill effects of free radicals (reactive oxygen species; ROS) within the body. Free radicals are produced as by-products of chemical reactions necessary to sustain life, for example, cellular respiration. Damage caused is dependent on the balance between the antioxidants and free radicals within the body. The influence of free radical scavengers (vitamins E and C, carotenoids and selenium) is significant and plays a role in the ageing process. Contributing to the development and/or exacerbation of a wide variety of degenerative diseases. Many factors can contribute to excessive levels of free radicals being produced. These include exposure to UV light and radiation, air pollution (including cigarette smoke), residues from herbicides and pesticides, and illness and the medications used to treat it. In some illnesses, patients in human medicine are actively encouraged to take antioxidants; these include those suffering from diabetes mellitus, arthritis and cancers.

TABLE 2.8 Functions of antioxidants in the body.

Antioxidant	Function
Vitamin A	Powerful anticancer and some antiviral properties. Helps maintain the stability of cell membranes.
Vitamin E	Protects polyunsaturated fatty acids (PUFAs) from peroxidation by free radicals.
Vitamin C	Regenerates vitamin E, glutathione and flavonoids.
Minerals (selenium, zinc, copper, iron and magnesium)	Selenium is linked with vitamin E. It is a coenzyme of glutathione peroxidase, acting as an antioxidant. The combined effect of vitamin E and selenium is more effective than either alone. High dietary concentrations of copper and iron may be pro-oxidants.
Alpha-lipoic acid	Helps to neutralise free radicals, can be used to treat nerve damage, and helps slow the development of ageing and cardiovascular disease.
L-Carnitine	When combined with alpha-lipoic acid (in a form known as acetyl-carnitine), the two substances have a synergistic effect and thus enhance particularly the anti-ageing and energy-producing properties.
Glutathione peroxidase	Dependent on selenium and glutathione for its formation. Especially important in reducing the production of inflammatory prostaglandins and leukotrienes.

PRE-, PRO- AND POSTBIOTICS

Prebiotics are substances that can alter the gastrointestinal flora in a manner that benefits the microorganisms. Probiotics are a live microbial feed supplement which benefits the host animal by improving the gastrointestinal microbial population. Probiotics generally used are comprised of lactic acid bacteria such as lactobacilli, streptococci and bifidobacteria. Probiotics are beneficial following acute gastroenteritis or a course of antibiotics, especially in hindgut fermenters such as rabbits and horses. Questions have been raised about the ability of the bacteria to survive the acidic environment of the stomach. Hence, the use of prebiotics has been stated to be more advantageous than probiotics. Probiotics, if administered, need to be provided in large enough numbers and potentially daily. Yeasts have also been included in some probiotic preparations. Their role is to aid in improving the digestibility of fibre and other nutrients. Populations of yeasts do not seem to be maintained within the established gastrointestinal flora, and thus, to maintain their effect, daily administration is required.

A postbiotic is a preparation of inactivated microorganisms, their components or byproducts that may have health benefits. Postbiotics can be used in food, supplements, and skincare products.

How do postbiotics work?

- Postbiotics can produce beneficial compounds like short-chain fatty acids, vitamins, amino acids and antimicrobial peptides.
- Postbiotics can help manage allergy symptoms by decreasing allergic reactivity.
- Postbiotics may help improve symptoms of inflammatory bowel disease (IBD), like Crohn's disease and ulcerative colitis.

Postbiotic uses

- Postbiotics can be used to reduce foodborne illness by targeting the farming stage of food production.
- Postbiotics may help manage allergy symptoms like runny or stuffy noses.
- Postbiotics may help improve symptoms of mild to moderate Crohn's disease and ulcerative colitis.

The three main mechanisms of action for probiotics are the following:

- Competitive Exclusion. Colonisation sites within the gastrointestinal tract and nutrients within the gut are utilised by the probiotics. This thus reduces the availability of resources to the potentially pathogenic bacteria. Chronic gut dysbiosis (when undesirable microorganisms take over in large numbers) can have detrimental effects on the immune system of the digestive system.
- Immunomodulation. A synergistic effect exists between probiotics and the stimulation and functioning of the immune system.
- Digestive efficiency. Probiotic microflora have an important role in aiding the breakdown of complex food nutrients.

Prebiotics are specific nutrients, which encourage the growth of beneficial bacterial populations (e.g. specific types of fibre). Benefits that the host will experience from this manipulation of the gastrointestinal bacteria include:

- Inhibition of potential pathogenic bacteria. This will cause a reduction in endotoxins, carcinogens and substances associated with putrefaction.
- Stimulation of gastrointestinal immunity.
- Increased synthesis of vitamins, especially B complex and K.
- Increased absorption of nutrients.
- Improved faecal consistency.
- Increased production of VFA/SCFA.

VFA benefit the animal by increasing available nutrients for gastrointestinal bacterial populations, which in turn aid in reducing the amount of nitrogenous waste materials entering the bloodstream and causing azotaemia. This process is sometimes referred to as nitrogen traps in renal diets. Examples of prebiotics include:

Manno-Oligosaccharides (MOS)

MOS are prebiotics that also aid in increasing the populations of certain microflora that benefit the animal. Its unique structure also attracts pathogens and bonds them to the manno-sugars, rather than attaching to the surface of the gut villi.

Glutamine

Glutamine is an amino acid commonly included in critical care nutrition diets due to its immune-enhancing properties and ability to enhance wound healing. Glutamine is utilised in rapidly dividing cells, like epithelial enterocytes and mucosal immune cells. Glutamine acts as a prebiotic by maintaining the overall health of the gut lining and therefore ensuring optimal nutrient absorption [3].

Fructo-Oligosaccharides (FOS)

FOS acts as a nutrient source for the beneficial bacteria of the GIT. FOS also increases gut transit time and draws water into the faeces, increasing bulk and softness.

NUTRIGENOMICS AND NUTRIGENETICS

Nutrigenomics and nutrigenetics are two complementary fields of nutritional genomics that explore the interaction between diet and genes. Nutrigenomics studies how nutrients, foods and diet patterns influence gene expression, studying how diet components (nutrients) affect gene expression (switching genes on or off). Nutrigenetics investigates how individual genetic variations (polymorphisms) affect the body's response to specific nutrients. Studying how an animal's unique genetic profile (polymorphisms/variations) causes it to react differently to specific dietary components.

REFERENCES

1. Michel, K.E. (2024). Nutritional assessment. In: *Small Animal Clinical Nutrition*, 6e (ed. M.S. Hand, C.D. Thatcher, R.L. Remillard, et al.), 554–555. Mark Morris Institute.
2. Moreno, A.A., Parker, V.J., Winston, J.A., and Rudinsky, A.J. (2022). Dietary fiber aids in the management of canine and feline gastrointestinal disease. *Journal of the American Veterinary Medical Association 260* (S3): S33–S45. https://doi.org/10.2460/javma.22.08.0351.
3. Perna, S., Alalwan, T.A., Alaali, Z. et al. (2019). The role of glutamine in the complex interaction between gut microbiota and health: a narrative review. *Int. J. Mol. Sci. 20*: 5232. https://doi.org/10.3390/ijms20205232.

CHAPTER 3

Energy Calculations

Calculations based on weight can ensure that the patient is receiving sufficient calories. The calculated energy requirement divided by the calorific value of the diet on an 'as-fed basis' will determine the quantity of diet to be fed. Daily weighing of the animal and using body condition scores (BCS) will confirm whether the calories provided to the animal are sufficient, adequate or excessive.

Basal Energy Requirements (*BER*) = the amount of energy required by a healthy animal in a thermoneutral environment, whilst awake but not exercising, 12 hours after eating.

Resting Energy Requirement (*RER*) = The RER differs from the BER as it includes energy expended for recovery from physical activity and feeding and is calculated from these equations, dependent on the weight of the animal. The RER for dogs and cats can be calculated with either of these two formulas:

$$\text{RER (kcal/day)} = 70\,(\text{BW}_{\text{kg}})^{0.75} \text{ (if body weight (BW) is less than 2 kg).}$$

or

$$30\,(\text{BW}_{\text{kg}}) + 70 \text{ (if BW is between 2 and 45 kg).}$$

It has been calculated that RER may be 1.25 BER, but many texts often regard the two as interchangeable values.

Maintenance Energy Requirements (*MER*) = the energy required for a moderately active adult in a thermoneutral environment. This includes energy for obtaining, digesting, and absorbing food in animals to maintain an optimal BW. The average values for a dog are 2 × RER and for a cat, 1.4 × RER.

Daily Energy Requirement (*DER*) = The DER represents the average DER for any animal, depending on life stage and activity. If the animal is in the home environment, we would use DER to calculate the energy requirement. The DER is calculated from the RER and a life stage factor.

Kitten (Growth) = 2.5 × RER
Neutered cat = 1.2 × RER
Entire cat = 1.4 × RER
Active cat = 1.6 × RER
Obese prone = 1.0 × RER
Weight loss = 0.8 × RER
Pregnancy = 1.6 – 2 × RER
Lactation = 2 – 6 × RER (dependent on the number of nursing kittens).

Some food manufacturers market different types of foods for neutered male and neutered female cats. There is a metabolic difference between the two sexes, but it is marginal.

Neutered dog = 1.6 × RER
Entire dog = 1.8 × RER
Obese prone = 1.4 × RER
Weight loss = 1.0 × RER
Active/working = 3 – 8 × RER
Pregnancy >21 d = 3 × RER
Lactation = 4 – 8 × RER (dependent on number of nursing puppies).

All calculations are rough estimates and should be adapted to the individual, depending on condition scores and weight gain and losses.

During weight loss programmes, the quantity of food is often reduced until weight loss is achieved. There is, however, a lower limit to the volume of energy that can be provided.

- Minimum amount that can be fed is 42.6 kcal/$TBW_{kg}^{0.75}$/day in dogs and 42.2 kcal/$TBW_{kg}^{0.711}$/day in cats

All animals must undergo a nutritional assessment to give good clinical advice regarding nutrition based on their requirements. Nutritional assessments are based on visual observations, such as BCS and muscle condition scores (MCS), but also on specific measurements such as weight, plasma protein measurements and other blood constituents (Figures 3.1–3.3).

When calculating a BCS for an individual, the animal must be visibly assessed and palpated. Use of the BCS index is the method of choice and can give an estimated figure for the ideal BW. There are BCS based on a five-, seven- or nine-point scale; the nine-point scale has been validated, so this should be the one of choice. Some breeds do not suit some aspects of the BSC index. For example, Whippets and Greyhounds in good condition have limited fat cover. The use of an MCS (Figure 3.4) should be utilised alongside the BCS. It is especially important to use the MCS when initiating a weight loss diet, as dramatic losses could be due to a drop in muscle mass and need to be prevented.

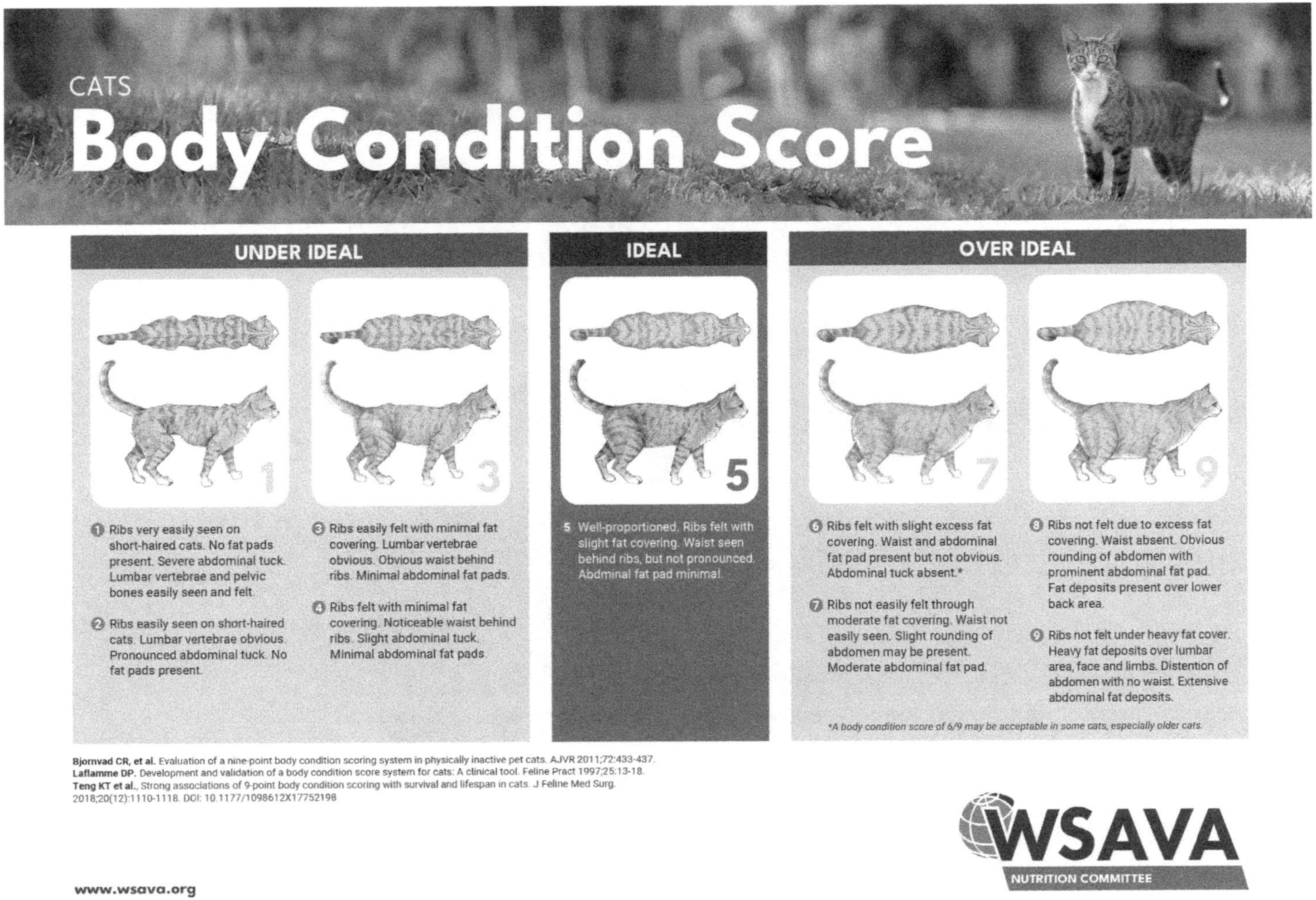

FIGURE 3.1 Nine-point body condition scoring system. With permission of Nestlé Purina PetCare.

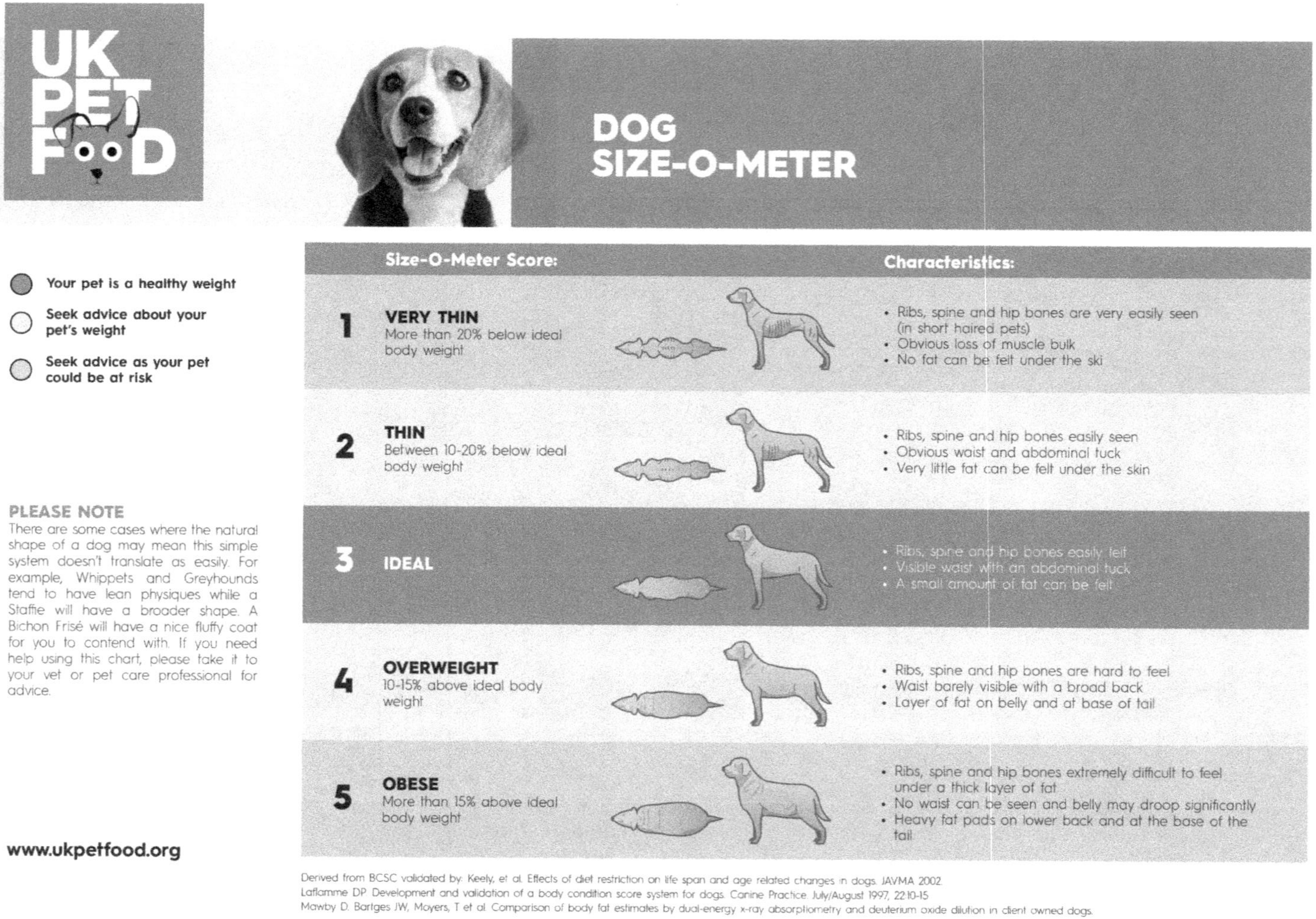

FIGURE 3.2 Five-point body condition scoring system.

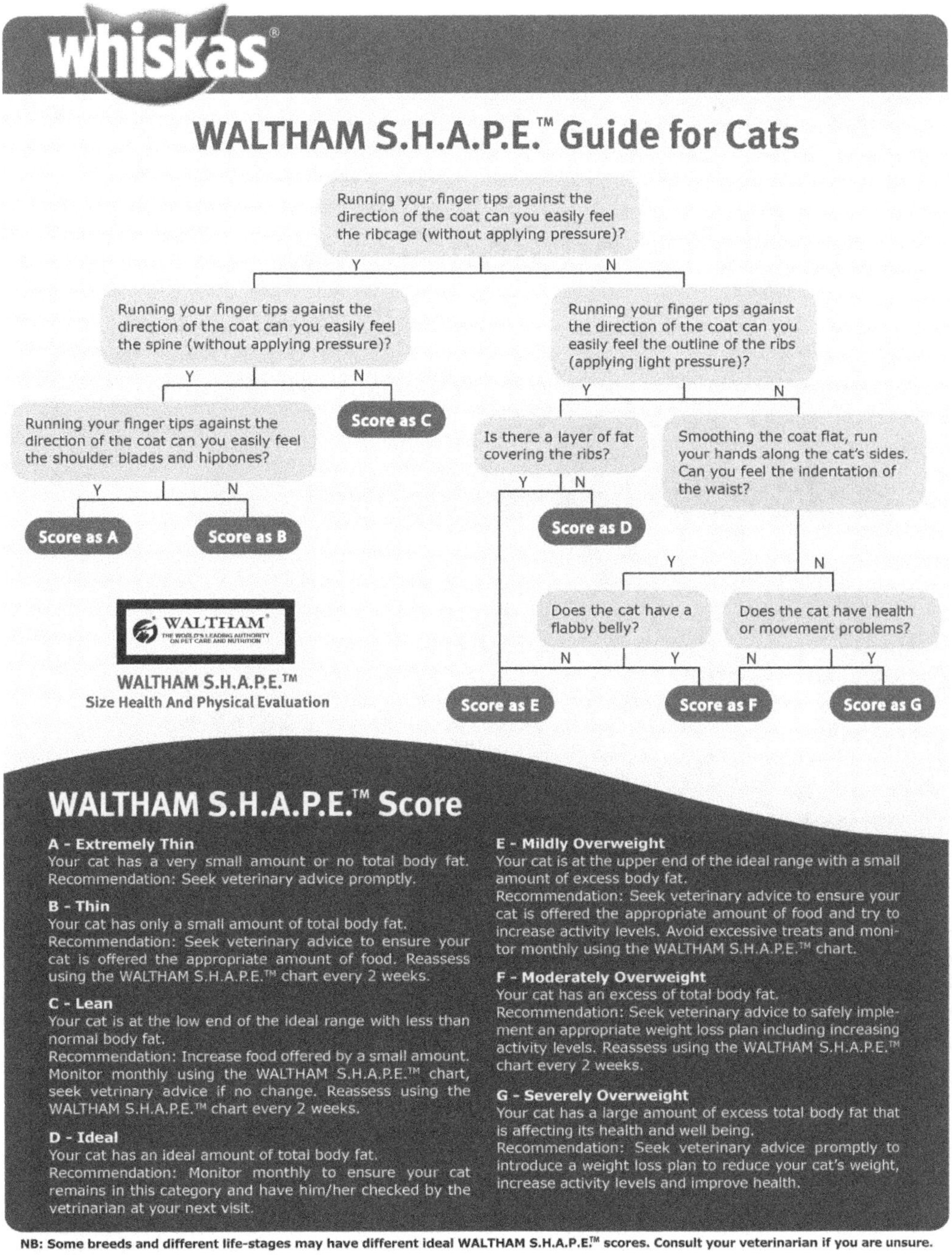

FIGURE 3.3 Waltham shape guide: seven-point body condition score system.

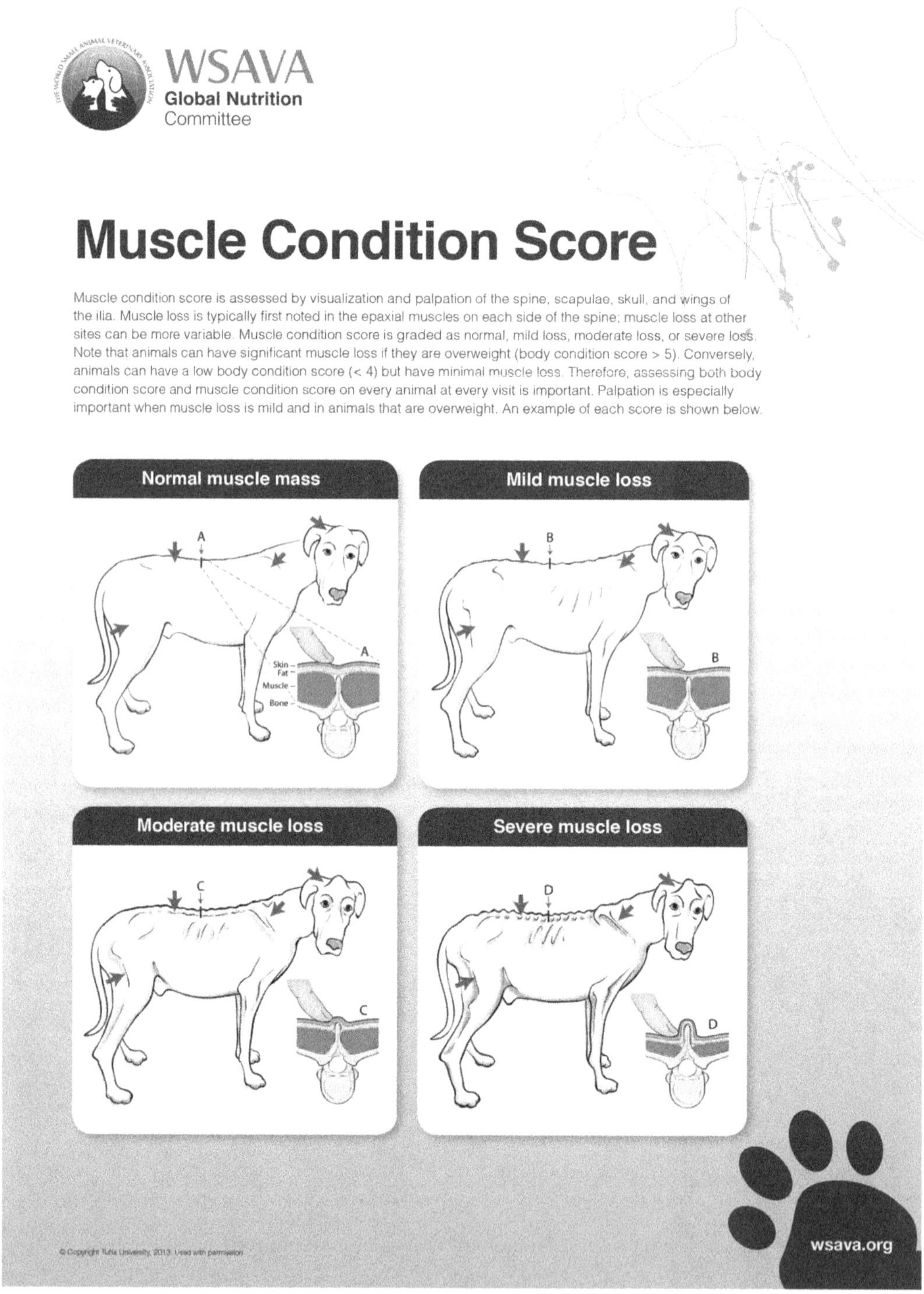

FIGURE 3.4 Muscle condition scoring system for cats. WSAVA (2020) / `https://wsava.org/wp-content/uploads/2020/01/Muscle-Condition-Score-Chart-for-Cats.pdf` / last accessed August 03, 2026.

MUSCLE CONDITION SCORING AND MONITORING MUSCLE MASS

Current methodology for monitoring muscle mass is through palpation, as described by the WSAVA Nutritional Assessments.

https://wsava.org/wp-content/uploads/2020/01/Muscle-Condition-Score-Chart-for-Cats.pdf.

Ultrasonographic measurement of feline epaxial muscle height (EMH) at the 13th thoracic vertebra (T13) is a repeatable, accurate, and non-invasive, point-of-care method for assessing muscle mass and sarcopenia. It is highly useful in wellness exams to detect early muscle loss (sarcopenia) that might not be visible.

Key Aspects of Monitoring EMH:

- **Technique:** The measurement is taken at the T13 level, where the ultrasound probe is placed to measure the distance from the vertebral-rib junction to the muscle–subcutaneous fat interface.
- **Accuracy:** Measurements are reliable across observers (both trained and untrained), making it a practical clinical tool for assessing sarcopenia, especially in senior cats.
- **Clinical value:** EMH positively correlates with BW and is a reliable, objective, non-invasive method for quantifying muscle mass changes over time.
- **Application:** It is used as part of annual wellness exams to detect early, subtle muscle wasting in mature and senior cats.
- **Measurement metrics:** The mean EMH is typically measured, but sometimes a ratio to the T4 vertebra length (VEMS – Vertebral Epaxial Muscle Score) is calculated to normalise for body size.

'Overcoat syndrome' occurs when an MCS of 1 or 2 is present, but the animal is carrying excessive amounts of subcutaneous fat. The large fat deposits mask the muscle wastage (sarcopenia) that is occurring. This can easily occur in animals that suffer from a dramatic decrease in food consumption, for example, acute anorexia. Other aspects of the physical examination of the patient should be taken into consideration. These aspects include hair coat quality and skin condition, evidence of peripheral oedema or ascites (which may indicate hypoproteinaemia) and clinical signs that indicate certain deficiencies in micronutrients (e.g. neck ventroflexion or tetany).

The use of BCS and MCS has be proven to be very useful with patients suffering from chronic conditions that can affect weight and body condition. Patients suffering from cardiac conditions can develop ascites; this fluid collection can cause an overall gain in BW. The patient's BCS and MCS, however, can decrease as lean body mass is lost. This highlights the importance of monitoring BCS alongside weight at each consultation.

Monitoring Nutritional Interventions

Once an animal has been recommended a specific dietary regime, the animal should be reassessed after an appropriate time. This does depend on the animal, severity of disease (if any present), original nutritional status and the type of nutritional intervention received. Regular weighing of the animal, BCS, MCS and, if possible, blood

TABLE 3.1 Percentage overweight using body condition scoring.

Body condition score	Percentage over/underweight
4–5	Ideal
6	10%
7	20%
8	30%
9	40%

haematology and biochemistry parameters can all be utilised in these cases. Animals that are placed onto diets that alter urinary parameters, for example, pH, should have these parameters monitored regularly.

Animals that are hospitalised should be weighed at least twice daily, and depending on clinical health, this may be required to be performed more often. All medications and fluid therapy flow rates are based on BW, and if the animal is severely dehydrated, as the animal is rehydrated, dose rates will need to be adjusted accordingly.

Calculating Ideal Body Weight

There are many recommendations regarding the calculation of an individual's ideal or optimal weight. Recording the animal's weight and BCS as a puppy or kitten and throughout the growth phase allows monitoring of the animal's body condition. Many practitioners take the animal's weight, which was recorded at the time of the first annual vaccination (~1 year old) as the individual's ideal weight. This can be a true reflection, but if the animal was overfed during the growth phase, this weight will be an overestimation. Likewise, in larger breeds, maturity and full adult size would not have been reached, and the use of this weight will be an underestimation of ideal BW. The use of breed guidance charts is not advised as there can be huge variations within breeds and they do not take into consideration frame size. When calculating an ideal BW for an individual, the animal must be visibly assessed and palpated with the use of a BCS (Table 3.1). Advising an owner what their animal should weigh, if never seen before, is not recommended.

Once an animal is obese on either of the body condition scoring systems, reference to the Hill's BFI chart will need to be made (Figure 3.5).

For example, if a dog weighs 23 kg and has been assessed at BCS9/9, the dog is 40% overweight. To calculate the ideal BW: current weight divided by 100% + percentage overweight, then multiplied by 100. In this example, $23/140 \times 100\% = 16.43$ kg.

ENERGY METABOLISM

The route by which energy (adenosine triphosphate, ATP) is obtained from the diet is dependent on the nutrients absorbed. Calculating the amount of energy from the diet that is ultimately metabolised by the body depends on digestibility and the amount of energy lost in urine and faeces and the energy required to absorb the nutrients (Figure 3.6).

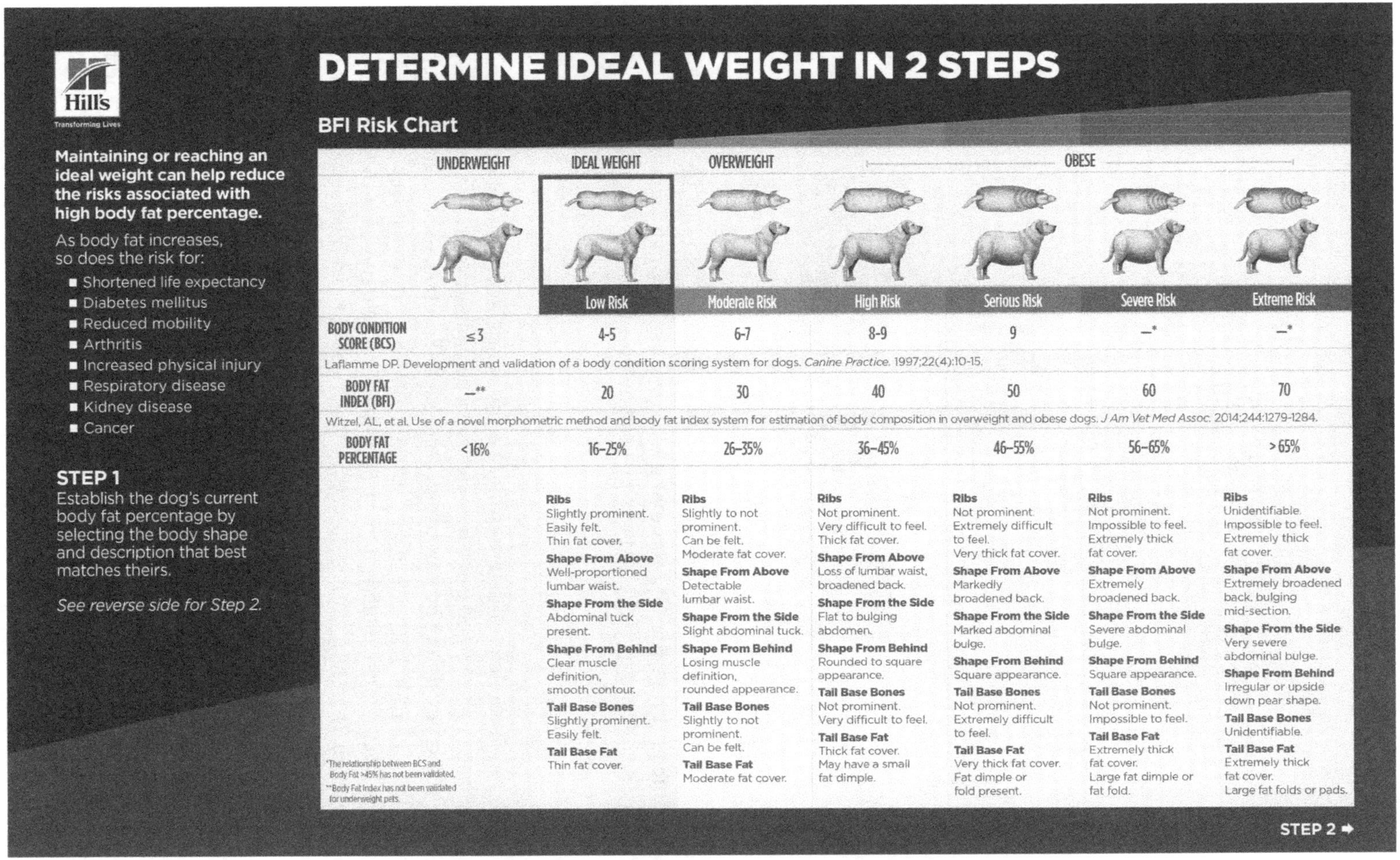

FIGURE 3.5 Hill's pet nutrition body fat index (BFI) chart.

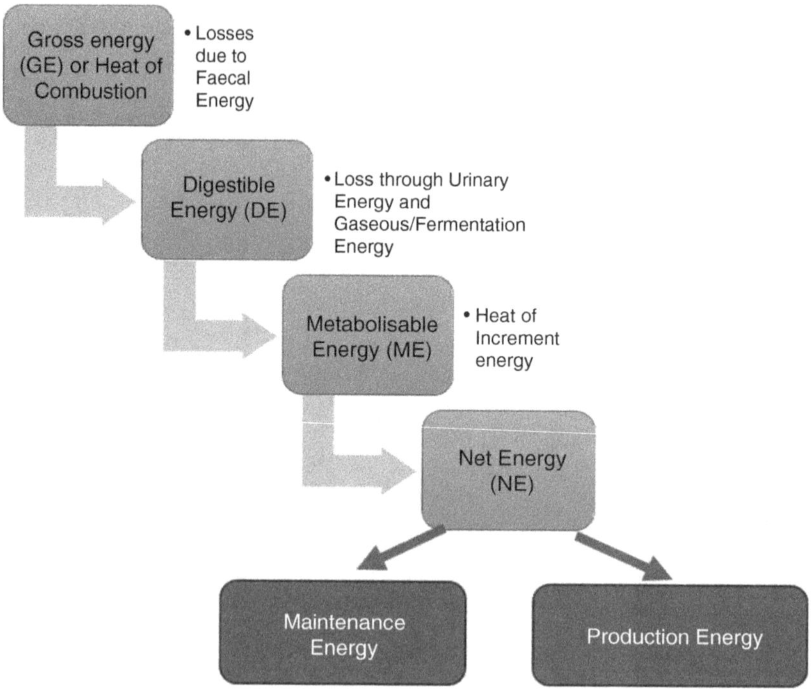

FIGURE 3.6 Energy flow through the animal.

The gross energy (GE) of the diet is the total heat produced by burning the food in a bomb calorimeter. From the GE, removing energies lost through incremental losses will result in the net energy (NE) that can be used by the animal.

Proximal Analysis of Food

The most common method of determining the nutrient content of the diet is through proximal analysis. This method calculates the diet's percentage of water (moisture), protein, fat, ash and crude fibre. The percentage that is left (i.e. 100% – % moisture – % crude protein – % fat – % crude fibre – % ash) is carbohydrates or nitrogen-free extract, NFE. Crude protein levels are calculated on the basis that the protein contains 16 ± 2% nitrogen. The crude protein, therefore, equals nitrogen × 6.25, or nitrogen divided by 0.16. Errors can occur when non-protein nitrogen such as urea or ammonia is used with the product. Figure 3.7 demonstrates the proximate analysis of foods.

Food Comparisons

The quality of the food cannot be assessed from the food label, especially the true digestibility of individual nutrients and the overall digestibility of the diet. The bioavailability of nutrients is not disclosed on the label, and this does need to be conveyed to owners when they compare foods. The typical analysis states the percentage of protein, oil (fat), fibre, ash and moisture (when over 14%). In the United States, a guaranteed analysis is used, where percentages are again used, but a minimum and a maximum value of each nutrient is given.

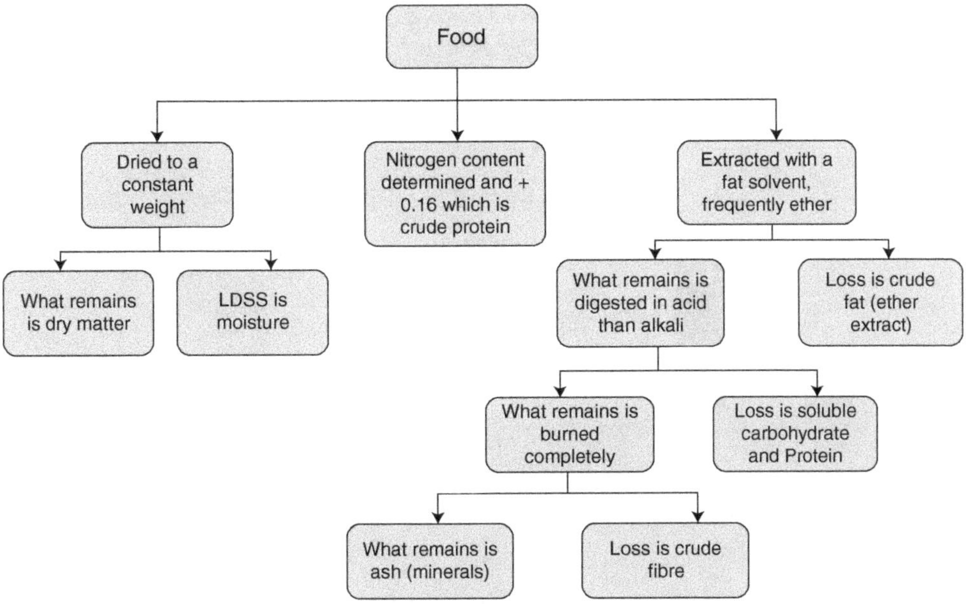

FIGURE 3.7 Proximate analysis of foods.

TABLE 3.2 Example of diet comparisons.

Phosphate content	Diet A	Diet B	Diet C
As fed	1.05%	0.84%	0.18%
Dry matter base	1.13%	0.91%	0.89%
Per 1000 kcal	0.3 g	0.3 g	0.35 g

The moisture content of the diet has a direct effect on the remaining ingredients. Moist diets are more dilute than dry diets. Thus, direct comparison of the typical analysis is inaccurate when moisture contents differ (Table 3.2). Comparisons should only be made when based on energy content (e.g. per 100 kcal).

Nutrient Percentages

All diets contain three main nutrients: fat, protein and carbohydrates. If we decrease one of these, for example, a protein-restricted diet like renal foods, one or both of the other nutrients' relative percentage has to increase (Figure 3.8).

Understanding this concept is vital and is what will help us with deciding on a diet for our animal.

Nutrient Recommendations

Each disease or disorder process has nutritional recommendations; as previously discussed, a reduced or restricted protein content in the diet could indicate an increase in the level of fat within the food. For example, for an animal suffering from renal disease and pancreatitis, a renal food wouldn't be ideal. Renal diets have restricted protein

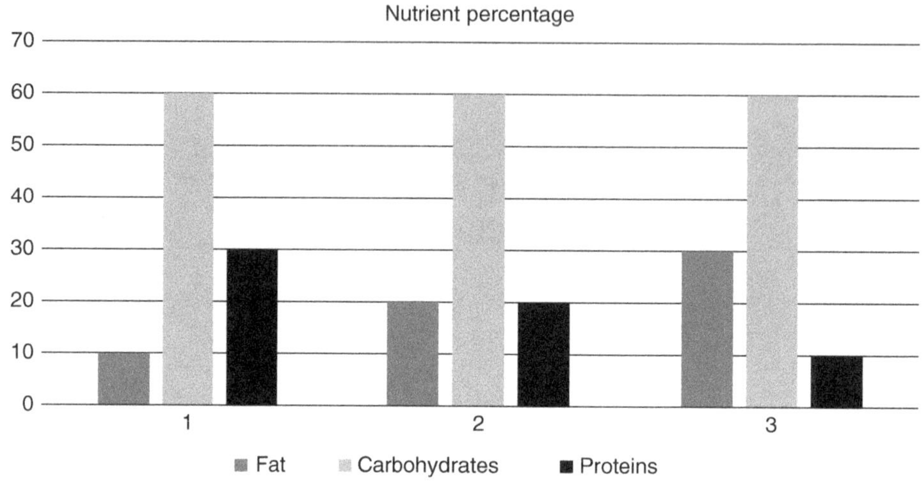

FIGURE 3.8 Relative percentages of nutrients in the diet. If the protein is decreased, as in Diet C, the fat content is increased.

TABLE 3.3 Comparison between dry and moist diets when calculated on a DMB.

Food A: 75% moisture, 10% protein
Amount of dry matter (100 – 75) = 25% dry matter
Protein content = 10/25 × 100 = 40% protein on DBM
Food B: 20% moisture, 10% protein
Amount of dry matter (100 – 20) = 80% dry matter
Protein content = 10/80 × 100 = 12.5% protein on DMB
Thus, Food A contains over three times as much protein as Food B on a DMB

DMB = Dry matter basis.

and, therefore, increased fat content; for pancreatitis, a high-fat diet isn't desirable. Ideally, a low-fat diet with the lowest phosphate content would be most suitable for this patient.

Comparing Diets

Comparing diets can be difficult; we need everything to be on a level playing field. We can't compare ingredient lists, 'As fed' or per dry matter basis (DMB), as we may need to feed more of one diet than another based on the calorific density of the diet.

In this example, if we used As Fed to compare, Diet C has the lowest phosphate content, but this is a wet food and ~80% water, so it skews the nutrient levels. Let's take the water content out and compare it on a DMB. Again, the diet with the lowest phosphorus content would be Diet C. However, when we calculate the content per calorific density, we have to feed much more as it is lower in calories, and, therefore, overall, you end up feeding much more of the other nutrients, such as phosphates. Diet A or B contains the least amount of phosphates.

Comparing the diets needs to be done on 'per 1000 kcal' or 'per 100 kcal'; make sure that you check that the energy densities are the same. If researching diets online, ensure you have the product that is produced for your country (Table 3.3).

CHAPTER 4

Food and Feeding

TYPES OF PROPRIETARY DIETS

Proprietary diets are those which are commercially made, that is, processed, and fall into two basic categories – complementary or complete.

Complete Diets

Complete diets are those that provide a nutritionally balanced and adequate diet when fed as the sole source of food. All of the nutrient components are provided in the correct ratio for the specific life stage and do not require any additions from any other food source. Adding other food sources to the diet in large quantities can make the overall daily intake of food nutritionally unbalanced. If any food rewards are to be given, the recommendation is that no more than 5–10% of the total daily energy requirement be in the form of treats.

Complementary Diets

Complementary diets are those which do not provide a nutritionally balanced diet when fed alone. These diets are designed to be fed in combination with other diets to form a balanced and adequate diet. All treats and snacks are labelled as complementary foods and thus should only make up a small portion (5–10% maximum) of the daily ration.

HOME-MADE DIETS

It is still relatively common for cats and dogs to be fed home-made diets. If prepared well and careful consideration has been made to ensure that it is balanced, home-made diets can serve some purpose in certain cases, for example, in food trials. Many home-made diets contain excessive quantities of protein and carbohydrates and are limited in vitamins and minerals, especially calcium. If owners do wish to pursue the use of a home-made diet, examples of a diet should be obtained from the veterinary practice. It is also advisable that the animal has its BCS, weight, and clinical health examined regularly to ensure that the diet is balanced and no deficiencies are present. Aiding the owner in designing the diet is important, and there are six simple guidelines to follow when designing a diet [1]. They are:

1. Do the five main food groups appear in the diet?
   - A multivitamin.
   - A source of minerals, including trace minerals, careful consideration should be made of calcium levels.
   - A fat source.
   - A protein source: it is vital in feline diets that an animal-sourced protein is used.
   - A carbohydrate source, which also includes fibre. Sources used should be from cooked cereals, grain or potato (potatoes and tapioca are excellent carbohydrate sources when performing food trials, as they are not commonly used in commercial diets).
2. What is the quality and source of the protein?
   - The protein levels and the protein quality within the diet are two very different elements. A high protein level does not necessarily mean that the animal is receiving all of the necessary essential amino acids (EAAs) it requires. Skeletal muscle protein from different sources does contain similar amounts of amino acids, and there is, therefore, no great advantage to feeding one type of meat over another. Unless it is for food trials. Novel protein sources used include duck, venison, salmon and egg. Egg is an excellent protein source (BV 100%), and in cases where restricted protein levels are required, the inclusion of egg as a protein source in the diet is highly recommended, as you ensure a high protein quality.
3. What is the fat content of the protein source?
   - Cuts of meat vary greatly in their content of fat. Where the fat content is high in the meat source, other fat levels may need to be reduced to compensate for this.
4. What is the carbohydrate-to-protein ratio within the diet?
   - The carbohydrate/protein ratio should be approximately 1:1 to 2:1 for cat diets and 2:1 to 3:1 in canine diets [1].
5. Is there a source of vitamins and minerals?
   - A home-made diet will potentially be unbalanced, and the supplementation of vitamins and minerals can be utilised. When using home-made diets for food elimination trials, the use of supplements is not recommended, as this will affect the trial. As the trial is not long-term, short-term deficiencies can be tolerated in many cases.
6. Is there a source of other essential nutrients?
   - Other essential nutrients such as essential fatty acids (EFAs), taurine and other EAAs may need to be supplemented into the diet to ensure adequate levels. This can be achieved through the addition of oils and other supplements.

Home-made diets should be cooked, as this aids in increasing the overall digestibility of the diet and reduces the risk of food poisoning. Overcooking will result in a loss of nutrients from the diet, especially vitamins and the denaturing of proteins. There are a vast number of different home-made diets available on the internet, and they can even be designed for a specific animal and/or clinical disease. Utilisation of the board-certified veterinary nutritionist would be the primary recommendation or use of specific software to formulate a home-made diet.

PALATABILITY

The palatability of any diet is essential if the animal is to consume it. The palatability of a food is its degree of acceptance by an animal. There are three essential components to palatability: the pet (species and individual), the environment (owner, home and lifestyle), and the food itself (smell, shape, texture, taste and nutritional composition). The first component, the pet, cannot be altered to enhance the palatability of the diet. The second component, the environment, can be changed in some ways. The habits of the owner around feeding time, the designated areas in which the animal is normally fed, the types of bowls used, etc., can all be changed to benefit the animal. Guidance from the veterinary practice should be available to be sourced by the client to aid the animal. The third component, the food itself, plays the largest role in palatability and will be discussed further.

Food Aroma and Temperature

The temperature of the food does play a huge role in the acceptance of the diet. Cats, in general, prefer food that is near body temperature. This is a direct reflection of their natural diet in the wild. Food that is taken straight from the fridge can be less appealing, as with foods above 40°C/104°F [2]. Though there will always be individual differences with each animal, trailing different food temperatures is recommended. Animals with dental pain or uraemic mouth ulcers may prefer cold foods. The aroma of the diet plays a significant role in the animal's acceptance of the food. Those animals that have a reduced olfactory capacity, such as older animals, sick animals and those on medications which reduce olfactory senses, can have a marked decrease in the acceptance of the diet. Cleaning any mucus from the animal's nose will aid in this. The use of moist diets can be advantageous; this is due to these diets giving off stronger aromas.

Prehension

How the animal picks up the food in its mouth and how it eats it have a role in the palatability of the diet. Cats exhibit three different methods of dry food prehension. The most common method is labial prehension. In this method, the cat grasps the kibble between the incisors without the use of the tongue. The second method, supralingual prehension, involves the cat using the dorsal side of the tongue to lap up their kibbles. The third method, sublingual prehension, occurs when the cat applies the ventral side of the tongue to the kibble, turning the kibble backwards into the mouth

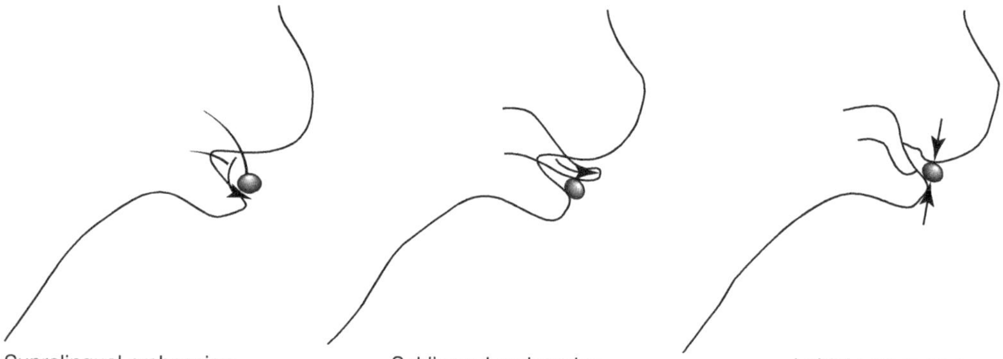

FIGURE 4.1 Diagram showing different methods of prehension.

(Figure 4.1). Sublingual prehension is commonly used in brachycephalic breeds, such as Persians. Different kibble shapes have been shown to suit certain types of prehension. For example, almond-shaped kibbles are best suited for cats, which use sublingual prehension.

Prehension and kibble shape and size do not seem to be linked in the dog. The kibble shape and size do affect other feeding parameters. Including the time taken to eat the diet and aiding in encouraging the dog to chew the kibble rather than swallowing it whole.

Taste

Once the animal has smelt the aroma of the food and picked it up into its mouth, taste is the third stage in food selection and a factor that affects the palatability of the diet. Taste perception can be modulated by four factors:

1. Sex: It has been found that female dogs are more receptive to sweet tastes than males. In many species, pregnancy and hormonal imbalances can also affect taste and responses to taste and smells.
2. Age: Taste sensitivity does decline with age.
3. State of health: Some diseases do affect taste. These include chronic renal failure, diabetes mellitus, thyroid dysfunction and cranial trauma. Nasal discharges will also affect the ability to taste, hence the requirement to bathe nasal discharges away to help cats suffering from viral infections to eat.
4. Drugs: For example, tetracycline alters taste perception.

The taste of the diet can be directly influenced by many factors, including the ingredients used, manufacturing practices, storage, pet food preservation systems, packaging and palatability enhancers.

Texture

The consistency of the diet does have large effects on the quantity fed, the palatability (in some cases), how the diet is stored and packaged, and the methods in which the animal is fed. Cats and dogs prefer meat-based canned products rather than dry expanded diets [3]. This has been attributed to the higher moisture content and due to blood and fluids containing positive palatability factors [3].

Moist Diets

Moist diets contain 70–85% moisture and are extremely popular. Packaging for moist diets can range from cans to foil trays and pouches. These diets are very palatable and can lead to overeating and obesity if the animal is allowed to have unlimited food. The moisture content of these diets can prove to be invaluable when trying to increase the water content of the animal's diet, especially in cases of FLUTD. It is recommended that all cats have a portion of their diet made up of moist foods.

Semi-moist Diets

Semi-moist diets contain around 30% moisture. The diet pieces are formed by the ingredients being cooked and formed into a paste. The paste is then passed through an extruder and shaped. Acid preservatives are then added to inhibit bacterial and fungal growth. Corn syrup or equivalents can be used to coat the pieces to prevent drying out and remove the availability of moisture for bacterial and fungal growth. The coating of the syrup makes the pieces very palatable but unsuitable for diabetic patients. Semi-moist diets should not be fed to cats as they can have the potential to contain propylene glycol as the coating. Propylene glycol is an approved food additive for dog food under the category of animal feed and is generally recognised as safe for dogs. Similarly, propylene glycol is an approved food additive for human food as well. `http://en.wikipedia.org/wiki/Propylene_glycol`. The exception is that it is prohibited for use in food for cats.

Dry Diets

The moisture content of dry diets can widely differ with estimates of between 6% and 12%, and can be made by several different methods. Using a mixture of dry flaked and crushed cereals and vegetables creates meal-type diets (Figure 4.2). These diets can be beneficial when catering for large numbers of animals, as each animal's requirements can be met; this is a common method for feeding horses. Forming the ingredients into a paste and cooking creates extruded diets. This process involves steam and pressure cooking. The cooking process can improve the digestibility of the diet, as some nutrients are broken down in the process. The extruded kibbles can then be coated in flavourings and packaged once dried.

Extruded diets tend to be complete and balanced for the life stage that they are designed for. In some species, extruded and pelleted diets are preferred as they prevent selective feeding, a common problem in meal-type diets, especially in rabbits and small rodents. Extruded diets do increase chewing compared to pelleted diets. Thus increasing palatability, increasing positive eating behaviour, no gulping, etc. This eating behaviour also causes an increase in the production of saliva. Extruded diets are ideal for working/performance diets for any species, as higher fat levels can be utilised.

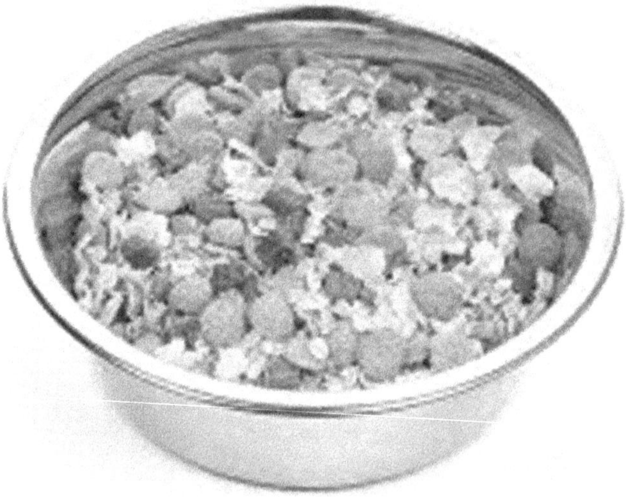

FIGURE 4.2 A mixture of dry flaked and crushed cereals and vegetables creates meal-type diets.

Some food manufacturers use a combination of extruded kibbles alongside semi-moist kibbles, as the semi-moist kibbles can aid in increasing the overall palatability of the diet.

Raw Commercial Diets

Commercially produced complete and balanced raw diets are available and, in the United Kingdom, can be submitted to voluntary bacteriology testing. These diets can be stored in different forms depending on the manufacturing process. Some will need to be frozen and thawed before consumption; some will be cold-pressed (ingredients are chopped and formed into pellets and then pressed to remove all water); and some will be vacuum-packed.

Fresh Foods

Definitions

Fresh food refers to pet food made from whole ingredients that are minimally processed, usually via gentle cooking (steaming or sous vide) at low temperatures to retain nutrients.

Sous vide (French for 'under vacuum') is a cooking technique that involves sealing food in a bag and cooking it in a precisely controlled, low-temperature water bath, usually with an immersion circulator. This method ensures consistent, edge-to-edge cooking and maximum moisture retention for meats, vegetables and eggs.

Ultra-processed foods (UPFs) are industrial formulations manufactured from processed ingredients and additives (e.g. preservatives, emulsifiers and artificial colours) with little to no whole-food ingredients, designed for convenience and long shelf life. Examples include fizzy drinks, packaged snacks, reconstituted meat and ready meals. Diets high in UPFs are strongly linked to increased risks of obesity, cancer, cardiovascular disease, and type 2 diabetes.

Introduction

The owners' requirements for food to feed their pets have changed dramatically in the last 30 years, with owners' demand for texture-rich diets to enrich their pet's dining experience driving this trend. One survey of 2,181 pet owners showed 87% were highly bonded with their pet, and 53.1% of pet owners reported giving the same or a higher priority (43.7%) to purchasing healthy food for their pet rather than for themselves [4]. In the United Kingdom, the market is worth £200 million and growing at 10% each year [5] (the whole UK pet food market is £2.7 bn). In the United States, raw, fresh, and frozen pet food market is experiencing rapid expansion, with specific segments valued between $4.1 billion (raw) and over $18 billion (combined raw/fresh/frozen) as of 2025–2026, with the overall pet food market valued at $77 bn [6]. The market is driven by pet humanisation, with a high Compound Annual Growth Rate (CAGR) of 11–21% expected for fresh formats, aiming to reach up to $5 billion by 2027 [6]. Many people use food to emotionally bond with their pets and want to maximise their eating experience with highly palatable foods and diet variety. For the multitude of reasons discussed above, some pet owners want to feed their dogs an alternative diet, such as home-prepared, organic, perceived human-grade, mildly cooked/fresh, vegetarian/vegan or raw diets.

Health Benefits

Does eating fresh food have health benefits over other food types? There are minimal studies that compare different food types with others; the studies that have been conducted comparing fresh foods with commercial extruded diets are not comparing like with like. In the most recently peer-reviewed published paper, 22 healthy mixed-breed geriatric Alaskan sledge dogs were fed the extruded diet (control) for a four-month washout period before being transitioned into their respective treatment group. Group 1 continued to be fed the control diet, whilst Group 2 was transitioned to a fresh, human-grade food (treatment). Individual serum samples were collected at day 0 and months 1, 3, 6 and 12, with metabolomic profiling of serum samples being performed [7]. The fresh diet showed superior metabolomic profiles over the extruded diet, but the diets were not the same in nutrient content.

Other studies have looked at diet types and their effect on biomes – gastrointestinal and skin biomes. Healthy client-owned dogs (8) were fed a fresh diet for 30 days, then dry foods for another 30 days after a 4-day transition period. Results from this study showed that there was an increase in bacterium types and a change in their relative quantity when dogs were fed a fresh dog food compared to these same dogs fed dry pet foods. This study was the first of its kind and shed some light on how different pet foods impact the skin microbiome [8]. Again, the diets were not of the same nutrient content.

Gastrointestinal microbiomes and metabolites are greatly affected by the nutrients within the diet. Fibre types (prebiotics) are widely used for this effect. Investigating the different forms of diet processing/cooking/preservation is important. A study investigating the apparent total tract nutrient digestibility of frozen raw, freeze-dried raw, fresh and extruded dog foods and their effects on serum metabolites and faecal characteristics, metabolites and microbiota of healthy adult dogs found that dietary format may lead to great differences in nutrient digestibility and faecal characteristics, metabolites and microbiota [9]. When appraising this study, the nutrient content between the diets could vary greatly; for example the protein content on a dry matter basis (DMB) in the extruded diet was 24.61%, whereas in the freeze-dried raw food, it was 56.75%; almost double [9].

There are many studies looking at digestibility, stool quality, hair quality and many other aspects; the studies are comparing fresh with commercial extruded diets, but the diets don't have the same nutrient content. For comparisons and conclusions to be made over which processing and preserving process is more advantageous, we need to be comparing the same diet (ingredients and nutrient profile) with the only variability being the cooking process (fresh and made into extruded kibbles).

Conclusion

The UPF movement has highlighted the health risks of eating these foodstuffs that are classed as UPF. Health experts are recommending not to eat these foods; the extrapolation of this advice is easily seen in the veterinary health sector. The role of fresh diets has a definite place in the nutrition market; more research is needed (in all diets), with direct comparison being important.

With fresh diets being cooked, the bacterial load is different from raw diets; the health and safety implications are different. Fresh diets might serve as a safer alternative to raw feeding for those who don't wish to use extruded diets.

Post-ingestion Effects

Once consumed, the gastrointestinal tract provides many signals related to food ingestion. The distension of the stomach with food stimulates stretch and chemoreceptors. These receptors send vagal signals to the satiety centre. Both positive and negative feedback mechanisms are responsible for regulating food intake. Negative feedback mechanisms such as insulin, serotonin, leptin, neurotensin and glucagon appear to attenuate food intake. Daily administrations of leptin have shown to decrease food consumption and thus induce weight loss [10]. Positive feedback mechanisms include the activation of the autonomic system during eating. Opioid and dopaminergic neurons are involved in the stimulation of food intake and aid in the positive reinforcement of food intake.

FEEDING BEHAVIOURS

Finicky Feeding Behaviour

Fastidious or finicky eating behaviours can make a transition to a new therapeutic veterinary diet almost impossible. This commonly occurring eating behaviour is a human-caused problem, resulting from the animal's conditioned expectations for frequent changes in the food variety or flavour. Owners will often describe their pets as finicky eaters if they are viewed to be intermittent or slow eaters. This can, however, be due to the animal being overfed or the animal's autoregulation of food consumption. Assessment of the animal's body condition score will conclude whether or not the animal is consuming sufficient nutrients.

Behavioural modification of the animal to counteract this feeding behaviour is difficult, as it is reliant on the owner. Often, the owner is the cause of the initial problem. Removal of the excessive rotation of different brands and flavours to less frequent changes may help resolve the problem. A ritualising feeding routine will need to be implemented, with set meals at a certain time, place and brand of food. Some animals that do self-regulate may benefit from ad libitum feeding. This does tend to be for small-breed dogs, as owners tend to overestimate the amount of diet that the dog can consume at any one time. With free-choice feeding, it is important that the overall daily amount of diet is still weighed out and supplied to the pet and that overconsumption of calories doesn't occur.

Those animals, which have been fed a high-quality, very palatable diet on an ad libitum basis (mainly cats), will expect this unlimited food availability. To change the animal's diet, it must be made to become dependent on the owner for food. To accomplish this, the animal should be offered ad libitum feeding for two set hours per day. Once this routine has been established, the old diet should be restricted to 75% of the previous food intake, and the rest of the daily requirement made up with the new diet, placed in a separate bowl next to the old diet.

Food Addictions

Food addictions are fairly common, for example, cats becoming addicted to tinned tuna. Addictions can lead to nutritional deficiencies or even toxic syndromes. Counter-conditioning behavioural modifications are required over some time. This modification can occur by adding a distasteful substance to the food, which the animal is addicted to, whilst providing a balanced, complete diet of the same flavour as the addicted food.

Food labels should be scrutinised as foods that are 'flavoured' are different from ones that contain that specific food ingredient. A prime example is tuna-flavoured cat foods that do not necessarily contain tuna.

FOOD AVERSIONS

The implications of food aversions are dramatically underestimated in veterinary practice. In some regards, it is not advisable to institute dietary changes whilst clinically ill patients are hospitalised. Diets should be introduced in the home environment once the pet is more stable.

The prevention of malnutrition by ensuring adequate nutrient intake is crucial in the management of all medical and surgical cases. The veterinary nurse or technician is crucial in practical measures to improve adequate intake. These practical measures include:

History Taking

Talking to the owner can prove to be invaluable. Obtaining information on preferred types and consistency of food, and the animal's eating habits, will contribute towards getting the animal to eat. Cats can be exceptionally fastidious concerning the size, shape and type of bowl or saucer that they eat out of. Wide-rimmed bowls tend to be preferred so that they have room for their whiskers.

Removal of the Clinical Problem

Many medical problems, for example, renal dysfunction, can result in changes in appetite and olfaction. Pain associated with dental disease or neoplasia in the mouth will also decrease appetite. Removal of pain or the causal agent will greatly improve the well-being of the patient.

Odorous Foods

Warming of the diet to body temperature can prove to be more appetising to the animal. Increasing the temperature will also increase the odour of the food. The use of highly odorous foods such as pilchards can aid to stimulate eating. None of these measures will work, however, if the animal is unable to smell the food. Any nasal discharges need to be cleaned away before offering the food.

Positive Reinforcements

Positive reinforcements such as hand feeding can be used to promote eating. Improving the animal's general well-being, for example, grooming, can also aid in this process. Trying to encourage eating outside the practice environment can prove to be useful. Taking small quantities of food when exercising the animal outside or feeding in a room away from all other animals might encourage the animal to eat. Timid animals can benefit from having somewhere to hide away in.

Food aversions can be reinforced by repeatedly offering a diet that the animal keeps refusing. Force-feeding should not be used to aid encouragement to eat, as the animal can become easily distressed, and this can cause a negative reinforcement to eat that particular food. Any offered food that is not consumed should be removed from the animal's environment after 15 minutes. Littering the animal's cage with a carpet of different foods will not encourage eating behaviours.

FEEDING METHODS

The method in which an animal consumes its diet does have an impact on many different elements of its life. There are four basic methods of feeding cats and dogs: free choice, ad libitum, time limited, or food limited. All have their advantages and disadvantages and will suit different animals on an individual basis. Significant breed differences have been noted in dogs and their feeding behaviours. Beagles and very small-breed dogs have similar feeding patterns to cats, whereas poodles are said to prefer eating only during the night-time hours. There are, however, always individuals who are exceptions.

Free-Choice and Ad Libitum Feeding

Ad libitum feeding does tend to suit those animals that will eat only what is required to meet their energy requirements. Overconsumption can easily lead to obesity, and in growing large and giant breed dogs, it can predispose them to developmental orthopaedic disorders (DODs). The animals are allowed to eat as much as they want throughout the day with no limits on volume. Other disadvantages include food wastage, especially if feeding a moist diet, and competition from other animals in the environment, which can lead to overeating and consequently under-eating in other animals. Advantages include a more constant blood level of nutrients and hormones and a decrease in coprophagy. Those animals that are timid are more likely to eat, as there is a longer period of access to the food, in which the other animal is not present to eat in front of. Many of these dogs tend to carry kibbles to a different site away from the main bowl of food and then consume them. This method of feeding is advised with animals with or predisposed to FLUTD. This is due to the postprandial alkaline tide; see the section on FLUTD for more details. With free-choice feeding, a fixed amount of diet is available to the animal, and they can choose when to eat. Once that daily fixed amount has been consumed, no more if offered.

Time-Restricted Meal Feeding

In this method, the animal is allowed free access to the food for a set period each day. This is usually 10–15 minutes, once or twice daily. This can be a disadvantage in small dogs, puppies, and kittens due to their limited stomach size, as insufficient food is consumed to meet their nutritional requirements. Overconsumption can easily occur when using this feeding method if the animal is greedy. In these cases, reducing the amount of time that the animal has access to the diet or feeding a diet of a lower energy density is required. Advantages include aiding in house-training puppies. A routine of feeding a puppy and then taking it outdoors can enforce house-training by taking advantage of the gastrocolic reflex.

Food-Restricted Meal Feeding

This method requires either calculating the DER of the animal and thus the quantity of diet that needs to be fed or following the manufacturer's recommendations on the food packaging. The calculated DER is then divided by the energy density of the diet to obtain the quantity of food that should be fed. The advantage of this diet is that when using a complete balanced diet, the animal is receiving the correct amount of nutrients. The disadvantage is that all animals are individuals, and when initiating this feeding method, a reassessment of the quantities fed should be made because some animals have a higher metabolism or workload and require higher amounts of energy. In these cases, a performance diet could be beneficial. Likewise, some animals may gain weight using this method, and in these cases, a lower energy-dense diet could be recommended.

Methods to Increase Water Consumption in Animals

Increased quantities of water within the diet are required for certain clinical diseases or disorders. Encouraging an animal to increase its consumption of water can be difficult, and several different methods may be required to achieve sufficient quantities consumed.

Cats

Cats can be extremely fastidious in what, when, and where they eat or drink. To increase water consumption, the availability of water needs to be increased. This can be achieved by placing more water bowls around the cat's environment (both inside and outside the house), using different types of water. Tap water, which is chlorinated, smells even more so to a cat. Allowing the water to stand for some time can remove a large portion of the chlorine and make it more palatable to the cat. Cats that live in a multi-cat household can find eating and drinking alongside other cats very intimidating. Making food and water available in a place where the particular cat feels safe can benefit them. The water content of the diet should also be increased; this can involve changing the cat over to a moist diet or adding water to a moist diet. Cats do not tend to consume dry biscuits that have had water added to them. The volume of water required to be added to make the diet more like a moist diet would render the food unpalatable.

The role of water fountains in increasing water consumption is widely advocated, but there is individual variation. If cats already like running, moving water, they will prefer the use of a fountain. Those who don't will not be encouraged to use one. Understanding the preferences of the cat is important to what is recommended.

Dogs

Encouraging dogs to drink more fluids can be easier in some cases than in cats, along with increasing the availability of water to the dog and allowing the water to stand for some time. The use of flavoured waters can tempt some dogs, but be careful of brands that are high in sugar. Ice cubes can also be used and are especially useful in hot temperatures. Stocks can be useful but have the potential to contain large amounts of salt. Low or zero-sodium stocks can be obtained.

Rabbits

Encouraging a rabbit to drink more fluids is very difficult but can be achieved. Thought should be given to the type of water container that the rabbit drinks from, whether the rabbit prefers a bowl or a water bottle. The use of grasses and hays, which have either been soaked or are wet, can be advantageous. Spraying the grass with water before putting the rabbit out can help increase water consumption.

REFERENCES

1. Tefend, M. and Berryhill, S.A. (2006). Companion animal clinical nutrition. In: *Clinical Textbook for Veterinary Technicians*, 6e (ed. D.M. McCurnin and J.M. Bassert), 438–492. Missouri: Elsevier Saunders.

2. Bourgeois, H., Elliott, D., Marniquet, P. et al. (2004). The influence of food characteristics on palatability. Focus Special Edition: dietary preferences of dogs and cats. 23–36.
3. Morris, J.G., Rogers, Q.R., and Fascettis, A.J. (2000). Nutrition of healthy dogs and cats in various stages of adult life. In: *Small Animal Clinical Nutrition*, 4e (ed. M.S. Hand, C.D. Thatcher, R.L. Remillard, and P. Roudebush), 529–562. Missouri: Mark Morris Institute.
4. Schleicher, M., Cash, S.B., and Freeman, L.M. (2019). Determinants of pet food purchasing decisions. *Can. Vet. J.* 60: 644–650.
5. Harmonic Finance. The UK Pet Food Market in 2024: ≈£4.1 bn overview (industry commentary). https://harmonicfinance.com/insight/an-appetite-for-change-the-uk-pet-food-market-in-2024/
6. TBRC Business Research Pvt Ltd (2026). Pet raw food market report: analysis of competition and future outlook. https://www.einpresswire.com/article/893338608/pet-raw-food-market-report-analysis-of-competition-and-future-outlook.
7. Ryan Yamka, Rae Sires, Joe Wakshlag, Heather J. Huson 2025. Serum metabolomics of senior dogs fed a fresh, human-grade food or an extruded kibble diet. *Metabolites* 15, 10, 676. https://doi.org/10.3390/metabo1510067
8. Kennedy Leverett, Rodrigo Manjarín, Erica Laird, Diana Valtierra, Tasha M Santiago-Rodriguez, Renan Donadelli, Gerardo Perez-Camargo 2022. Fresh food consumption increases microbiome diversity and promotes changes in bacteria composition on the skin of pet dogs compared to dry foods. *Animals 12*, 1881. https://doi.org/10.3390/ani12151881
9. Oba, P.M., Templeman, J.R., and Swanson, K.S. (2024). Apparent total tract nutrient digestibility of frozen raw, freeze-dried raw, fresh, and extruded dog foods and their effects on serum metabolites and fecal characteristics, metabolites, and microbiota of healthy adult dogs. *Transl. Anim. Sci.* 8: txae163. https://doi.org/10.1093/tas/txae163.
10. LeBel, C., Bourdeau, A., Lau, D., and Hunt, P. (1999). Biological response to peripheral and central administration of recombinant human leptin in dogs. *Obes. Res.* 7 (6): 577–585.

CHAPTER 5

Lifestage Nutrition

LIFESTAGE DIETS OF DOGS AND CATS

Gestation and Lactation

Recommendations state that prior to breeding, the bitch or queen needs to be in good condition. This includes nutritional status, that vaccinations are up to date, and that any parasiticide agents are administered (endo- and exo-parasiticides). An ideal body condition score (BCS) and muscle condition scores (MCSs) are required. Bitches and queens that are overweight could present with dystocia during parturition. Obesity, as demonstrated in humans, can also affect fertility. Maintaining bitches during the first six weeks of pregnancy on their original adult diet is possible, provided that the diet is of good quality and is not lacking in any specific nutrients. During the final trimester, the bitch will need to be switched to a growth/puppy diet. Large-breed puppy diets are not recommended even for large-breed bitches. These dogs will require a puppy growth diet for dogs under 25 kg. This is due to large-breed puppy diets having a decreased level of energy, which is especially required by the bitch in the last three weeks of pregnancy. The bitch's weight should increase to approximately 25% more than that at the time of breeding; this does depend, however, on the number in the litter. During this stage, more frequent feeding may be required due to a decrease in the quantity of diet consumed at each meal. If the bitch is having difficulties consuming adequate calories, free-choice feeding should be introduced. Fresh water must be made available at all times. Any reduction in water intake will dramatically affect milk letdown and the amount produced by the dam or queen.

The feeding of queens during pregnancy does differ to that of dogs. Queens increase food intake soon after conception, and this increases with the duration of gestation. During the first third of pregnancy, the queen will lay down fat reserves, which will be used towards the end of gestation and during lactation.

Lactation places huge stress on the nutritional demands of the bitch or queen. The nutritional demands can increase from 3 to 6 times that of maintenance. This is dependent on the number in the litter. The growth diet still needs to be fed free choice (rather than ad libitum) so that volumes can be monitored. Large volumes of water will be required and must be available at all times, as a decrease in water intake can affect milk production. Peak lactation demands will occur at three–six weeks of age, and further nutritional support of the bitch and queen will be required. Colostrum is vitally important to all mammals; it contains many antibodies from the bitch or queen, aiding in the early immunological status of the puppies or kittens. Queens and bitches can sustain a loss of body weight during lactation. Ad libitum feeding during pregnancy will allow for the increase in body tissue that will be metabolised during lactation and to meet foetal energy demands. The weaning body weight of the queen or bitch should not be less than the body weight at conception. Continual monitoring of the body weight of the bitch or queen, alongside BCS, is important to ensure that adequate energy is being consumed.

When nursing, puppies and kittens should be vigorous and active. For the first three–four weeks with puppies and four weeks with kittens, exclusive feeding from the mother is possible if she is healthy. The expected weight gain of kittens should be 10–15 g/day and puppies 2–4 g/day/kg of anticipated adult weight (or at least 10% gain per day). Puppies and kittens that are not receiving sufficient milk will cry, become restless or exhibit extreme inactivity and fail to achieve the expected weight gain. It should be remembered that littermates would differ and gain weight at different rates. This can be much greater in cats, where a litter may be sired by different Toms.

Hand-Rearing Puppies and Kittens

The most obvious alternative to being reared by the mother is by a foster mother. If this is not possible, hand rearing is the other alternative. Many puppy and kitten formulas are available, and each has specific feeding guidelines. The calorific needs for most nursing-age puppies and kittens are 22–26 kcal/100 g BW. The quantity of daily feedings is dependent on the formula guidelines, but the formula should be warmed to 37.8°C (100°F) before each feeding.

All equipment, bottles, teats, etc., need to be sterilised before feeding. In most cases, it is more convenient to prepare a 24-hour supply of milk and divide this into portions required for each meal. The prepared formula must be stored in a refrigerator; any unused prepared formula should be discarded if not used within 48 hours. Chilled prepared formula should not be fed to a puppy or kitten without warming, as colic can be induced. Once fed, the abdomen should appear enlarged but not over-distended.

Tube feeding is another method of feeding orphaned puppies or kittens. If a suckling reflex is present, bottle-feeding is the preferred method of choice due to fewer potential complications, like aspiration. When tube feeding, the formula should be warmed and administered over two minutes. This will allow sufficient time for the slow filling of the stomach.

After feeding, stimulation of the anogenital area is required. This is normally performed with warm, moist cotton wool. This provokes the reflex of micturition and defecation. By three weeks of age, puppies and kittens are usually able to relieve themselves without simulated stimulation.

Worming regime of the bitch and queen and of the litter must be implemented and will have a large effect on the nutritional status and well-being of all. This is due to the transmission of the parasites, *Toxocara canis*, transplacentally and transmammally. In the queen, worming is only required post-partition as *Toxocara cati* is only transmitted transmammarily. Studies have shown that a good worming regime will result in larger, healthier puppies and kittens. The offspring will require worming fortnightly from two weeks of age until 12 weeks old.

Weaning

The idea of solids can be introduced to the puppies or kittens from three weeks of age. A mixture of the mother's diet mixed with warm water is ideal. At this age, the puppies and kittens will show an interest and taste the food but will not be consuming enough to meet nutritional requirements. Observing the mother eating the diet is important and will encourage the puppies or kittens to start lapping. When eating their first solid food, kittens do not choose the most palatable food according to innate criteria. They will choose what their mother eats, even if their food is unusual. From six to eight weeks of age, complete weaning can start and be achieved. In the majority of cases, the bitch or queen will wish to spend less time nursing and may start to get annoyed or frustrated at them when they try to suckle.

On weaning, puppies and kittens need to be fed a good-quality complete growth diet. Advising new owners on a correct diet is vital. Questions about the diet need to be asked by veterinary practices on this subject when the new puppy or kitten is initially presented at the practice. Many breeders that use complete growth diets will rehome with the recommendation that the animal remains on the same diet during this transitional period. There is no reason to change the diet unless the animal isn't gaining weight adequately, if the diet isn't nutritionally balanced, or if the animal is grossly overweight.

Feeding Puppies and Kittens

Puppy growth diets are divided into those designed for pups, which will be greater than 25 kg when full-grown, and those that will be less than 25 kg when fully grown. This division is due to growth rates and the age at which maturity is reached. Large breeds should grow at a slower rate over a longer time. Diets designed for these breeds are modified with lower energy levels, thus preventing rapid growth rates. Historically, these large breeds' diets were supplemented with calcium, as it was felt that extra calcium was required to support the skeletal system during the rapid growth rate. Extra calcium is not required and should be kept in the ratio of 1:1 to 1.5:1 with phosphorus. If the energy content of the diet is correct, rapid growth phases are prevented, and the predisposition of developmental orthopaedic disorders (DOD) is reduced. DODs are discussed in more detail in the clinical nutrition section.

Overfeeding in all puppies and kittens should be avoided, as it can lead to obesity in later life. Slight underfeeding, which does not induce a reduction in full growth potential, will aid in increasing the animal's lifespan. Despite this, high-energy-dense diets are required in growth diets due to the limited capacity of the stomach and thus the quantity of food able to be consumed in each meal. Differences in the sizes of individuals within the litter can be due to many factors, including different fathers, so encouraging a more rapid weight gain for any smaller individuals should not be advocated as these individuals may just be smaller.

Assessment of weight gain needs to be performed on a daily basis for the first few weeks of life. Once weaned and rehomed (normally at eight weeks), puppies and kittens (eight to ten weeks) should be weighed at least fortnightly until three months and then monthly until six months old. This does conveniently fit in with the required worming regime. The use of growth charts can be invaluable and will enable trends in weight gain to be monitored. Too slow a weight gain can reflect insufficient calories being consumed or that the diet's protein quality is not adequate.

Addition of treats into the diet increases greatly during this phase of life, as socialisation and training in puppies occur. Using some of the pup's complete diet kibbles can be helpful, as it will prevent unbalancing of the diet and can help stop bad feeding habits from being formed. Advice on healthy treat options and other methods of positive reinforcement, that is, use of toys, social interaction and playing, should be relayed to the owner. The setting up of good feeding habits and behaviour occurs at this age, and puppies and kittens should be introduced to these from an early age.

DHA has been shown to improve cognitive ability and visual acuity and has been introduced into commercial puppy and kitten diets. Due to its benefits, DHA has the potential to speed training, obedience and socialisation.

Junior and Adolescent Diets

Some commercial dog foods do offer a junior or adolescent choice. The role of these diets can be beneficial in puppies that require an intermediate diet before moving on to an adult maintenance diet. For those brands that do not provide a large-breed puppy diet, utilising this junior/adolescent diet is necessary to prevent rapid growth rates. When large-breed puppy diets are being fed, changing to a junior or adolescent diet is not required as large-breed puppy diets have a reduced energy content compared to puppy diets.

Adult Maintenance

The adult phase is defined from when maturity has been reached until physiological changes occur due to the ageing process. The age at which the adult phase starts depends mainly on breed variations. Smaller breeds can reach full maturity from six months, and larger and giant breeds from one year to 18 months. Each animal should have their diet altered to meet the individual's needs. The quantity of diet fed will depend on the quality of the diet fed, the amount of exercise the animal receives, neutering status and metabolism. Those breeds which are predisposed to weight gain should have their weight, BCS and MCS monitored throughout this life phase. Changes of metabolism post-neutering (including chemical castration methods) should be noted to owners, and use of 'light' diets or diets specifically aimed at neutered animals should be advocated. These diets are designed to prevent weight gain and do not aid in weight loss.

Neutered Adult Diets

Many diets have now been introduced to the market, specifically designed for neutered animals. As previously discussed, after neutering, the animal's metabolism does decrease. In entire cats, energy expenditure in both female and male animals is 57 ± 2 kcal/kg. Once neutered, this value decreases to 50 ± 3 kcal/kg in males and 51 ± 2 kcal/kg in females. There are, however, marked differences in other factors as demonstrated in Table 5.1. Changes in insulin resistance can suggest a predisposition of neutered cats to diabetes mellitus.

Performance and Working Diets

Animals, which have a high-energy expenditure, will benefit from a diet which has a higher energy density. Due to the stomach's limited capacity, insufficient quantities of the diet may not be consumed if the dog has a reduced appetite or if time working/exercise limits the time available in which to consume the diet. The digestive system's capacity and digestive and absorption abilities can be a limiting factor. Care should be taken during periods of reduced activity levels, as excessive calories will result in quick weight gain. High-energy-dense diets are also beneficial for these animals that have a high metabolism and thus find weight gain difficult. When changing any animal to a high-energy-dense diet, a longer-than-normal transitional period may be required. This is due to the dog's

TABLE 5.1 Difference between male and female cats and the consequences of neutering.

Parameter	Male	Female	Consequence of neutering
Body fat (as % of total body weight)	23.8 ± 1	30.1 ± 1.7	Increase M: 32.9 ± 1.7 F: 35.5 ± 1.8
Energy expenditure (kcal/kg)	57 ± 2	57 ± 2	Decrease M: 50 ± 3 F: 51 ± 2
Nonesterified fatty acids		Higher in females	Greater differences between males and females.
Caloric requirements			Requirements were reduced in both sexes.
Serum leptin	Regulation of leptin secretion by testosterone	No demonstrated oestrogenic control in cats	M: Increase in males. F: Less noticeable change.
Glucose intolerance		Absent	Unchanged in both sexes.
Insulin	More marked		Continuance of high insulin resistance in males. Whereas in females, the appearance of insulin resistance.

digestive mechanisms having to adjust to this diet. The extra energy required in these diets is supplied in the form of increased fat content whilst having a decrease in fibre content. This increase in fat content is due to the increase in calories per unit of weight the fat contains. The reduction of fibre is required, as this will increase the digestibility of the diet and reduce the effect that fibre has on reducing the absorption of other nutrients.

Breed-Specific Diets

Many commercial diets are now aimed at specific breed types or sizes. Small-breed diets tend to have a higher energy density compared to those aimed at medium and large breeds. This is due to the small capacity of the stomach and an increase in metabolism. Care should be taken for those small-breed dogs, which put on weight easily, and in some cases, small-breed diets might not be the diet of choice. Kibble size is also altered depending on the size and breed of dog for which it is designed. In feline diets, kibble shape has also been shown to affect the way in which certain breeds consume their diet. Persian cats benefit from an almond-shaped kibble due to the shape of their skull.

Diets aimed at reducing the risk of certain breeds' disposition to certain disorders/diseases have been introduced onto the nutritional market. Diets aimed specifically for Bedlington Terriers are now commonplace and have reduced copper levels.

Senior Diets

The nutrition of older cats and dogs can be complex and very dependent on the individual, and there is an argument that there is no one singular diet that could be recommended for all animals. A nutritional assessment should be performed on all patients at every appropriate point of contact. A nutritional assessment comprises weight, BCS, MCS and nutrition history (what, where, how they eat), including behavioural aspects as these are especially important.

Energy Requirements

The proposed nutritional requirements for senior cats were traditionally fewer calories (as they are more inactive in advancing ages), lower protein levels, softer kibbles and a reduction in sodium and phosphorus in the diet. It has been discovered that the energy requirements in cats do alter and can increase once geriatric stages are reached [1]. Different stages of senior life will require different energy requirements, alongside different disease processes, and a possible reduction in activity if osteoarthritis is present will also influence energy requirements. Recommendations are made that the nutritional assessment be undertaken to make the assessment of these energy requirements. In dogs, however, the energy expenditure does tend to decrease as expenditure from exercise decreases. With cats, the nutrient assimilation from the diet declines, as cats have a decrease in the digestibility of proteins and fats as they age. The metabolisable energy requirements for senior cats can be equal to or higher than those in growth phases.

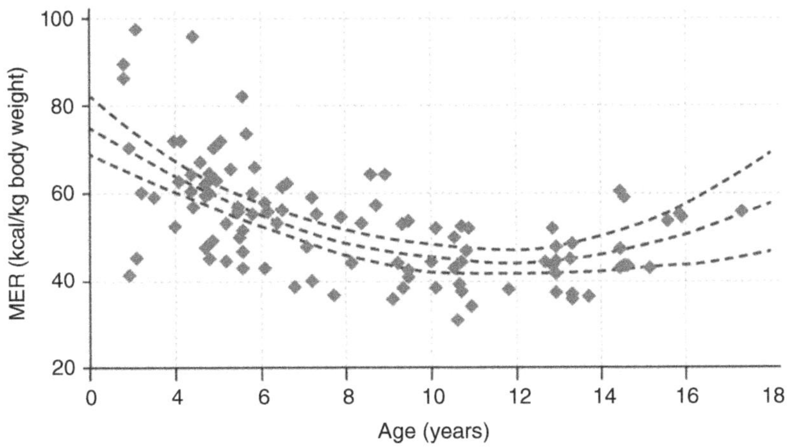

Studies have demonstrated an increased incidence of obesity with increased age up to 11 years, but after this peak, a loss of body mass, fat and lean tissue tends to be seen [2]. The speed of decline in body weight can be a predictor of mortality, with progressive decline in body weight reported in the 2 years prior to death [3].

Protein Requirements

A reduction in renal function should be considered in all senior animals; a reduction in protein quantities within the diet could be beneficial if renal damage has occurred [2]. The quality (the biological value) of the protein should be increased as skeletal muscle mass reduces, which also reduces any protein or amino acid reserves. Some lifestage diets do not have a decrease in protein levels, as restricted protein levels are not required until there is direct evidence of renal impairment [2]. Protein restriction in both feline and canine senior diets should be avoided. Cats are especially sensitive to decreases in protein levels within the diet. This is due to the inability to downgrade protein metabolism pathways. Reduced fat digestibility is also experienced in geriatric cats [3]. In healthy adult cats, protein digestibility is typically 85–90%. In geriatric cats, this digestibility can be reduced to less than 77%. Diets, which have a severely restricted protein level or proteins of a low quality/BV, can predispose cats over 12 years to negative nitrogen balance and loss of lean body mass [3].

The restriction of phosphorus in the diet does play a significant role in the prevention of renal impairment [4]. A decrease in kidney function can also lead to an increased loss of the water-soluble vitamins, due to the kidneys' decreased ability to concentrate the urine. This can also lead to a reduction in the hydration levels of the animal. Senior animals have a reduced sensitivity to thirst, and thus there is a greater risk of dehydration in these animals.

Water

Increasing water consumption can be achieved in a number of different ways: feeding a moist diet rather than a dry diet and by increasing the availability of water. Increasing the number of bowls (including types) around the house and allowing water to stand for a period of time prior to being offered to some animals can be beneficial. This allows the chlorine in the water to evaporate off, which some animals do prefer. Use of water fountains can also help to increase water intake. Ideally, phosphate-free hydration broths that can aid in increasing calorific intake alongside hydration without an increase in phosphate. As part of the nursing clinic, it is important to discuss with the client how to monitor hydration levels. Demonstrating monitoring of clinical signs can help the client in the care of their pet. This can include testing for skin tenting, tacky mucus membranes and the colour of membranes. If pet owners know what is normal, when the animal becomes unwell or the renal disease progresses, they can flag this to the practice more quickly. Ultimately, increasing the welfare of the animal.

As the animal ages, smell is the first sense to decline. As the animal's sense of smell deteriorates, the animal may eat less. The aroma of the diet is particularly important in diets aimed at senior animals to encourage consumption. Wet diets do smell more than dry, though it should be remembered that a cat's dietary preference is also based on the texture of the diet [5].

Diets supplemented with antioxidants, prebiotics and fatty acids had significantly higher average serum vitamin E levels and significantly better-maintained body weight and lean body mass, skin thickness and haematocrit values in comparison to cats on the control diet, as well as a more beneficial faecal microbiota balance. Overall quality of life did appear better but wasn't measured [6].

Medium-Chain Triglycerides (MCT)

There are now many senior diets that have medium-chain triglycerides (MCTs) supplemented within them. MCTs are a subgroup of fats converted to ketone bodies in the liver and are used as the preferential source of energy by cerebral cells. Long-chain triglycerides (the fats usually found in the diet) are utilised differently within the body. Supplementation with MCTs has demonstrated improved cognitive function in older dogs [7], although there are no effects that have been demonstrated in cats. A diet supplemented with a blend of 5.5% MCTs showed that there were improvements in trainability of dogs (with the ability to learn new tasks quicker), increased interactivity with others and interest in play, with improvements in alertness, compared to a control group [7]. These MCTs were obtained from the addition of coconut oils to the diet. This is thought to be due to the ketone bodies improving mitochondrial function, increasing polyunsaturated fatty acid content in the brain and decreasing amyloid precursor protein [8, 9].

Mobility

Osteoarthritis is a common radiographic finding in older cats and dogs, with a prevalence of up to 90% in appendicular joints (in both species) [10]. A randomised, controlled, double-blinded prospective clinical study examined a diet high in fish oil, green-lipped mussel extract, and glucosamine/chondroitin in client-owned osteoarthritic cats. The authors found that osteoarthritic cats receiving the diet, as compared with a control group, were more active as measured objectively with a collar-mounted accelerometer over a nine-week period [11]. Although this is not direct evidence of improvement, it was theorised that increased activity reflected decreased pain associated with OA.

FIBRE AND THE MICROBIOME

Many manufacturers of senior diets don't raise the importance of dietary fibre. The animal itself cannot digest soluble fibre in the diet, but the microbes within the intestine can. Soluble fibre is fermented into short-chain fatty acids (SCFAs) or volatile fatty acids (VFAs). These products are an important energy source for the intestinal cells and can increase blood flow to the intestine.

Nitrogenous waste products in the blood are presented to the intestinal lumen, where urease, an enzyme produced by intestinal bacteria, hydrolyses the urea into ammonia and carbon dioxide. The ammonia is then utilised by the intestinal bacteria. This process means that nitrogenous waste products are excreted in faecal matter, rather than in urine, by the kidneys. Dietary fibre may also be beneficial for improving gastrointestinal motility and colonic transit times. This is debated due to a decrease in the overall mobility of the animal, a potential decrease in water intake or through nutritional changes.

Carnivore vs Omnivore

Both cats and dogs are formally classed as carnivores. The metabolism and nutritional needs of the dog do approach those of the omnivore classification. Dogs have the ability to synthesise taurine, arachidonic acid and vitamin A from the metabolic precursors cysteine, linoleic acid and beta-carotene, respectively. Vets, however, are obligate carnivores and require these specific nutrients in a preformed state from a meat-based diet.

Rabbit Lifestage Diets

Lifestage diets are now commonly available on the commercial market. All of these diets are designed to be complementary and fed alongside grass and hay. Rabbits need to have a low requirement for fat levels in their diets; 1–2% is ideal. Any fat within a diet needs to be of vegetable origin. Animal fats contain cholesterol that can cause the rabbit to develop atherosclerosis-like symptoms. A recommended protein level for an adult maintenance diet is 12–14%. Animals that require high energy levels due to physical, environmental and psychological stressors may require a protein level of 16–22%. A fat level of 1% and fibre content of 20% are often quoted. Changes in the way in which rabbits are now kept should be remembered. House rabbits are now commonplace, alongside neutering. Neutering has a similar effect on metabolism as it does in cats and dogs. Rabbit caretakers should be made aware of this, as obesity can occur, and prevention is better than cure.

There are many different opinions surrounding which vegetables are suitable for rabbits. The majority of sources agree with carrots, carrot tops, broccoli and parsley to be safe. Carrots are considered safe but should only be fed in small amounts due to the high sugar content. Other vegetables that have been used also include dandelions, turnip greens, spinach, kale and romaine lettuce. Beans, potatoes and some lettuces are potentially problematic. Recommended guidelines for the amount of vegetables given daily are to feed at least three types of greens daily (along with carrots, if wished to be fed). It is important to feed more than one type of vegetable to prevent nutrient imbalances. The use of a complementary pelleted diet can aid in reducing any imbalances down. Some vegetables do contain high levels of oxalates (kale, mustard greens and spinach); instead of removing them from the diet altogether as there are benefits, limit their use to 1–3 meals per week. If you are advising a rabbit caretaker (rabbit owners prefer caretaker) on increasing the vegetable content of the rabbit's diet, it is exceptionally important to make any changes slowly. Also, that vegetables are washed thoroughly before offering them to the rabbit.

Rabbits should not be fed high-sugar treats, that is, chocolate drops. Treats for rabbits do exist; examples include small amounts of dried foods. These must be fed in very small quantities, but in reality, the rabbits don't need them in their diet. Chocolate is poisonous to rabbits and should not be fed; yoghurt drops have very high sugar content. Other foods that should be avoided include pasta, bread, biscuits, crackers and breakfast cereals.

Young Rabbits

Alfalfa can be fed to young bunnies under the age of six months since it provides extra calcium and protein necessary for growing bones. It is important to offer timothy or meadow hays as well, so when it comes time to wean them to strictly grass hay, they will know the taste and be less likely to resist change. Pelleted lifestage diets tend to contain higher levels of alfalfa, and thus an increase in calcium and protein levels. Up to the stage of sexual maturity, which tends to be around six months of age, a diet containing 16–18% protein, 3% fat and 16–18% fibre is required in order to allow for growth and development.

Young rabbits are only fed once daily by their mother, as the mother's milk is exceptionally high in fat. Feeding in this manner will also reduce the risk of predators locating the nest. The young rabbits will start to be interested in solids at roughly two weeks of age and will consume what the doe is eating. The act of caecotrophy usually starts at around three weeks of age. A healthy mixture of greens, hay and pellets is recommended, as it will encourage the young rabbits to have a varied diet. Complete weaning occurs at five–sixweeks of age. When the young are rehomed, it is recommended that they are fed the same diet as when with the doe. Any dietary changes must occur very slowly; the stress of separation can also act as a factor in digestive upset. Once the young rabbit has completely settled in, any required dietary changes should be made.

Senior Rabbits

At present, there are no lifestage diets designed for older rabbits. The diet of these rabbits should reflect any clinical problems usually associated with older age. Weight loss commonly occurs, but the causative problem rarely does. In some cases, the use of alfalfa can be useful as it has a higher energy density and is slightly more enticing to eat than grass hay. Those animals with dental problems would benefit from vegetables cut slightly small or pellets moistened in order to aid in an adequate nutrient intake. In cases where the animal appears in pain, the use of analgesia should be highly recommended. In many cases, it is often ignored by the owner as a consequence of old age.

REFERENCES

1. Groves, E. (2019). Nutrition in senior cats and dogs: how does the diet need to change, when and why? *Companion Animal* 24 (2): 91.
2. Sparkes, A.H., Caney, S., Chalhoub, S. et al. (2016). ISFM consensus guidelines on the diagnosis and management of feline chronic kidney disease. *J. Feline Med. Surg.* 18: 219.
3. Taylor, E.J., Adams, C., and Neville, R. (1995). Some nutritional aspects of ageing in dogs and cats. *Proc. Nutr. Soc.* 54: 645.
4. Plantinga, E.A., Everts, H., Kastelein, A.M.C., and Beynen, A.C. (2005). Retrospective study of the survival of cats with acquired chronic renal insufficiency offered different commercial diets. *Vet. Rec.* 157: 185.
5. Pekel, A.Y., Mülazımoğlu, S.B., and Acar, N. (2020). Taste preferences and diet palatability in cats. *J. Appl. Anim. Res.* 48 (1): 281.
6. Cupp, C., Kerr, W.W., Jean-Philippe, C., and Patil, A.R. (2008). The role of nutritional interventions in the longevity and maintenance of long-term health in aging cats. *Int. J. Appl. Res. Vet. Med.* 6 (2): 69.
7. Pan, Y., Larson, B., Araujo, J.A. et al. (2010). Dietary supplementation with medium-chain has long-lasting cognition-enhancing effects in aged dogs. *Brit. J. Nutr.* 103 (12): 1746.
8. Studzinski, C.M., MacKay, W.A., Beckett, T.L. et al. (2008). Induction of ketosis may improve mitochondrial function and decrease steady-state amyloid-beta precursor protein (APP) levels in the aged dog. *Brain Res.* 21: 209.
9. Taha, A.Y., Henderson, S.T., and Burnham, W.M. (2009). Dietary enrichment with medium chain-triglycerides (AC-1203) elevates poly-unsaturated fatty acids in the parietal cortex of aged dogs; implications for treating age-related cognitive decline. *Neurochem. Res.* 34: 1619.
10. Kerwin, S.C. (2010). Osteoarthritis in cats. *Top. Companion Anim. Med.* 25 (4): 218.
11. Lascelles, B., DePuy, V., Thomson, A. et al. (2010). Evaluation of a therapeutic diet for feline degenerative joint disease. *J. Vet. Intern. Med.* 24: 1.

CHAPTER 6

Gastrointestinal Biome

PREBIOTICS, PROBIOTICS, AND POSTBIOTICS: MECHANISMS AND BENEFITS

Prebiotics are substances (nutrients) that can alter the gastrointestinal flora in a manner that benefits the microorganisms. Probiotics, however, are a live microbial feed supplement which benefits the host animal by improving the gastrointestinal microbial population. Probiotics generally used are comprised of lactic acid bacteria such as *Lactobacilli*, *Streptococci* and *Bifidobacteria*. Probiotics have been shown to be beneficial following acute gastroenteritis or a course of antibiotics, especially in hind-gut fermenters such as rabbits and horses. Questions have been raised about the ability of the bacteria to survive the acidic environment of the stomach. Hence, the use of prebiotics has been stated to be more advantageous than probiotics. Probiotics, if administered, need to be provided in large enough numbers and potentially daily. Yeasts have also been included in some probiotic preparations. Their role is to aid in improving the digestibility of fibre and other nutrients.

The three main mechanisms of action for probiotics are:

- Competitive exclusion. Colonisation sites within the gastrointestinal tract and nutrients within the gut are utilised by the probiotics. This thus reduces the availability of resources to the potentially pathogenic bacteria. Chronic gut dysbiosis (when undesirable microorganisms take over in large numbers) can have detrimental effects on the immune system of the digestive system [1].
- Immunomodulation. A synergistic effect exists between probiotics and the stimulation and functioning of the immune system.
- Digestive efficiency. Probiotic microflora have an important role in aiding the breakdown of complex food nutrients.

Prebiotics are specific nutrients which encourage the growth of beneficial bacterial populations (e.g. specific types of fibre). Benefits that the host will experience from this manipulation of the gastrointestinal bacteria include:

- Inhibition of potential pathogenic bacteria. This will cause a reduction in endotoxins, carcinogens and substances associated with putrefaction.
- Stimulation of gastrointestinal immunity.
- Increased synthesis of vitamins, especially the B complex and K.
- Increased absorption of nutrients.
- Improved faecal consistency.
- Increased production of volatile fatty acids (VFA)/short-chain fatty acids (SCFA).

VFA benefit the animal by increasing available nutrients for gastrointestinal bacterial populations, which in turn aids in preventing the quantity of nitrogenous waste materials from entering the bloodstream and causing azoteamia. This process is sometimes referred to as nitrogen traps in renal diets. Examples of prebiotics include:

Manno-Oligosaccharides (MOS)

MOS is a prebiotic that also aids in increasing the populations of certain microflora that benefit the animal. Its unique structure also attracts pathogens and binds them to the manno-sugars rather than attaching them to the surface of the gut villi [1].

Glutamine

Glutamine is an amino acid commonly included in critical care nutrition diets due to its immune-enhancing properties and ability to enhance wound healing. Glutamine is utilised in rapidly dividing cells like epithelial enterocytes and mucosal immune cells [1]. Glutamine acts as a prebiotic by maintaining the overall health of the gut lining and, therefore, ensuring optimal nutrient absorption [1].

Fructo-Oligosaccharides (FOS)

FOS acts as a nutrient source for the beneficial bacteria of the GIT. FOS also increases gut transit time and draws water into the faeces, increasing bulk and softness.

Postbiotics

Postbiotics are by-products of the digestion of probiotics and prebiotics, and they may have health benefits. They can include SCFA, vitamins, amino acids and more.

- Postbiotics are created when probiotic bacteria break down fibre from foods like fruits, vegetables, grains and legumes.
- Postbiotics can also be produced during the fermentation of organic nutrients.

Potential health benefits

- Postbiotics may help with:
  - Gut microbiota modulation

- Antioxidant activity
- Immunomodulatory effects
- Epithelial barrier function
- Infant colic
- Atopic dermatitis
- Diarrhoea

Examples of postbiotics

- SCFA, like butyric acid, acetic acid and propionic acid
- Vitamins B and K
- Amino acids
- Antimicrobial peptides
- Phenylacetic acid

Potential applications

- Postbiotics may be used to promote health and productivity.
- Postbiotics may be used to substitute antibiotics.
- Postbiotics may be used to improve health outcomes.
- Postbiotics may be used to revolutionise the food and animal product industries.

ROLE OF PROBIOTICS WITH ANTIMICROBIAL USE

Introduction

Probiotics have been widely used and recommended in people to lessen antimicrobial-associated gastrointestinal signs (AAGS) (Box 6.1), with occurrence rates of between 1% and 44%, rates seem to be dependent on the antimicrobial type administered [1, 2]. There is empirical data that shows the positive role of probiotics in lessening the potential of AAGS in people [3–5]. Adverse drug effects, which can include AAGS, can affect compliance in people; premature discontinuation of antimicrobials occurs in 6–60%

Box 6.1 Clinical signs of antimicrobial-associated gastrointestinal signs (AAGS)

Vomiting, nausea and drooling
Dysrexia (including anorexia, hyporexia and pica)
Abdominal discomfort and pain
Diarrhoea

of people due to AAGS [6–12]. With concerns around antimicrobial resistance (AMR) as part of the One Health initiative, completion of courses of prescribed medications is an important factor in veterinary medicine. The co-administration of a probiotic alongside antimicrobials has demonstrated a threefold decrease in AAGS in people [1, 2, 13, 14].

The administration of antimicrobials has been shown to cause disturbance in the microbiome, predominantly decreasing the diversity of organisms present [17, 19–22]. Adverse events, especially AAGS, have been noted in both cats and dogs, with a range of different antimicrobials, due to these disturbances in the microbiome [15–18]. Clinical signs from studies [15–18] have mirrored those in Box 6.1, with measurements of food intake (overall calorific intake) also showing to be significantly decreased in the administration of clindamycin in cats [15]. Though this study was the only one to measure calorific intake.

Decreasing Aags

The inclusion of probiotics has been investigated in both cats and dogs being co-administered with antimicrobials (clindamycin [15], amoxicillin-clavulanate [17], metronidazole [16, 18] and enrofloxacin [16]). All the studies showed positive clinical outcomes for groups receiving a probiotic or synbiotic alongside the antimicrobials compared to a placebo or control group. These studies also commented on the positive effects of the probiotics or synbiotics persisting from six weeks [15] to > nine weeks after discontinuation [16].

Clinical Significance

Co-administration of probiotics or synbiotics with antimicrobials can help with a decrease in AAGS. In turn, this can help in compliance with the administration of the antimicrobial course. Owners should be offered the inclusion of probiotics when prescribed antimicrobials, at the discretion of the clinician and case suitability. Administration of a probiotic/synbiotic combination one to two hours after [20] or two hours before [17] each antimicrobial dosage is warranted to minimise AAGS as well as derangements in the faecal microbiome and metabolome [20].

The role of probiotics and the gastrointestinal biome is an area of great interest; what has been limited evidence in smaller sample sizes is increasing in importance and potential in the veterinary field.

The hypothesis of 'postbiotics' is under process, and their associations with antimicrobials turn out to be a new insight in antimicrobial therapy. Postbiotics provide a great opportunity to understand the mechanism of action against pathobionts; on the other hand, they lead to the postulation of newer pharmabiotic products and pharmacological strategies for better gut health. Postbiotics refer to the metabolic by-products like enzymes, peptides, teichoic acid, peptidoglycan-derived muropeptides, exopolysaccharides, cell surface and secreted proteins, bacteriocins and organic acids generated by a probiotic organism during its lifespan [19, 21]. Probiotics are living organisms which eventually die, but they secrete these postbiotics as a nutritive patrimony that continues to improve health. Postbiotics avoid risks linked with the administration of live probiotic bacteria.

More research is required on the role of postbiotics in the veterinary field and when antimicrobials have been administered.

REFERENCES

1. McFarland, L.V. (2008). Antibiotic-associated diarrhea: epidemiology, trends, and treatment. *Future Microbiol.* 3: 563–578.
2. Lenoir-Wijnkoop, I., Nuijten, M.J.C., Craig, J., and Butler, C.C. (2014). Nutrition economic evaluation of a probiotic in the prevention of antibiotic associated diarrhea. *Front. Pharmacol.* 5: 13.
3. Wilkins, T. and Sequoia, J. (2017). Probiotics for gastrointestinal conditions: a summary of the evidence. *Am. Fam. Physician* 96: 170–178.
4. Rondanelli, M., Faliva, M.A., Perna, S. et al. (2017). Using probiotics in clinical practice: where are we now? A review of existing meta-analyses. *Gut Microbes* 8 (6): 521–543.
5. Guo, Q., Goldenberg, J.Z., Humphrey, C. et al. (2015). Probiotics for the prevention of pediatric antibiotic-associated diarrhea. *Cochrane Database* 4 (4): CD004827.
6. Llor, C., Hernández, S., Bayona, C. et al. (2013). A study of adherence to antibiotic treatment in ambulatory respiratory infections. *Int. J. Infect. Dis.* 17: e168–e172.
7. Pechere, J.C., Hughes, D., Kardas, P., and Cornaglia, G. (2007). Non-compliance with antibiotic therapy for acute community infections: a global survey. *Int. J. Antimicrob. Agents* 29: 245–253.
8. Chan, Y.H., Fan, M.M., Fok, C.-M. et al. (2012). Antibiotics nonadherence and knowledge in a community with the world's leading prevalence of antibiotics resistance: implications for public health intervention. *Am. J. Infect. Control* 40: 113–117.
9. Munoz, E.B., Dorado, M.F., Guerrero, J.E., and F.M. (2014). The effect of an educational intervention to improve patient antibiotic adherence during dispensing in a community pharmacy. *Aten. Primaria* 46: 367–375.
10. Kardas, P., Devine, S., Golembesky, A., and Roberts, C. (2005). A systematic review and meta-analysis of misuse of antibiotic therapies in the community. *Int. J. Antimicrob. Agents* 26: 106–113.
11. Jefferds, M.D., Laserson, K., Fry, A.M. et al. (2002). Adherence to antimicrobial inhalational anthrax prophylaxis among postal workers, Washington, D.C., 2001. *Emerg. Infect. Dis.* 8: 1138–1144.
12. Jafarnejad, S., Shab-Bidar, S., Speakman, J.R. et al. (2016). Probiotics reduce the risk of antibiotic-associated diarrhea in adults (18–64 years) but not the elderly (>65 years): a meta-analysis. *Nutr. Clin. Pract.* 31: 502–513.
13. Selinger, C.P., Bell, A., Cairns, A. et al. (2013). Probiotic VSL#3 prevents antibiotic-associated diarrhoea in a double-blind, randomized, placebo-controlled clinical trial. *J. Hosp. Infect.* 84: 159–165.
14. Guo, Q., Goldenberg, J.Z., Humphrey, C. et al. (2015). Probiotics for the prevention of pediatric antibiotic-associated diarrhea (review). *Cochrane Database Syst. Rev.* 12: CD004827.

15. Stokes, J.E., Price, J.M., and Whittemore, J.C. (2017). Randomized, controlled, crossover trial of prevention of clindamycin-induced gastrointestinal signs using a synbiotic in healthy research cats. *J. Vet. Intern. Med.* 31: 1406–1413.

16. Whittemore, J.C., Moyers, T.D., and Price, J.M. (2019). Randomized, controlled, crossover trial of prevention of antibiotic-induced gastrointestinal signs using a synbiotic mixture in healthy research dogs. *J. Vet. Intern. Med.* 33: 1619–1626.

17. Torres-Henderson, C.S., Summers, S., Suchodolski, J., and Lappin, M.R. (2017). Effect of Enterococcus faecium strain SF68 on gastrointestinal signs and fecal microbiome in cats administered amoxicillin-clavulanate. *Top. Companion Anim. Med.* 32: 104–108.

18. Fenimore, A., Martin, L., and Lappin, M.R. (2017). Evaluation of metronidazole with and without Enterococcus faecium SF68 in shelter dogs with diarrhea. *Top. Companion Anim. Med.* 32: 100–103.

19. Tsilingiri, K. (2012). Probiotic and postbiotic activity in health and disease: comparison on a novel polarised ex-vivo organ culture model. *Gut* 61: 2011-300971.

20. Whittemore, J.C. (2021). Effects of synbiotics on the fecal microbiome and metabolomic profiles of healthy research dogs administered antibiotics: a randomized, controlled trial. *Front. Vet. Sci.* 8: 665713. https://doi.org/10.3389/fvets.2021.665713.

21. Konstantinov, S.R., Kuipers, E.J., and Peppelenbosch, M.P. (2013). Functional genomic analyses of the gut microbiota for CRC screening. *Nat. Rev. Gastroenterol. Hepatol.* 10: 741–745.

22. Hempel, S., Newberry, S.J., Maher, A.R. et al. (2012). Probiotics for the prevention and treatment of antibiotic-associated diarrhea: a systematic review and meta-analysis. *JAMA J. Am. Med. Assoc.* 307: 1959–1969.

CHAPTER 7

Cancer

CLINICAL NUTRITION

Nutrition can play an important role in the 'prevention' and treatment of cancers. This does, however, vary with the type of tumour and stage of progression. The potential risk reduction of cancer when following dietary recommendations has not been well documented in veterinary medicine. In human studies, 'eating right', staying active and maintaining a healthy weight can reduce the risk of cancer by 30–40% [1]. It has been speculated that this reduction may be even more achievable in pets as their dietary intake can be more controlled. Correct feeding of the cancer patient can enhance the quality and length of life. This is due to nutritional support reducing or preventing toxicoses associated with cancer therapy and ameliorating cancer-induced metabolic alterations. Inappetence and anorexia are common clinical symptoms in cancer patients, which can lead to weight loss and cachexia in conjunction with metabolic alterations. The use of body and muscle condition scores can be an excellent monitoring tool to assess the overall nutritional effect of cancer and treatments. Cancer affects the nutritional status of the animal in three ways:

1. Therapy (e.g. chemotherapy-induced anorexia, nausea or vomiting). Human chemotherapy patients have reported changes in taste and smell. These side effects experienced during therapy make it difficult for some patients to consume an optimal quantity of calories and nutrients.
2. Alterations of the metabolic pathways.
3. Tumours can also have a primary effect such as compression or infiltration of the alimentary canal.

The aims of nutrition for these animals are to:

- Meet the increased nutritional requirements of the patient whilst providing an energy source that the tumour cannot readily utilise.

- Ensure sufficient calories and nutrients are being consumed to maintain lean body mass.
- Limit lactate production by the tumour.
- Improve immune function, remission and survival times.
- Aid in limiting tumour growth.

CANCER CACHEXIA

Cachexia is defined as a profound and marked state of general ill health and malnutrition. It is a complex paraneoplastic syndrome that includes progressive weight loss that occurs despite adequate nutritional intake [1]. Loss of both fat and muscle can occur with the depletion of muscle mass often exceeding that of the viscera in cancer patients. Cachexia is not common in veterinary cancer patients, but weight loss usually occurs early in the course of the disease. Cachexia can cause a decreased quality of life, a decreased response to therapies and shortened survival time when compared to those with similar diseases without cachexia. Cancer cachexia may be partly due to a negative energy balance (Figure 7.1). It is therefore important for the owner to have the animal weighed and body condition scored regularly.

Carbohydrates

The metabolism of carbohydrates is greatly altered in dogs with cancer. The alteration in metabolism is due to tumours metabolising glucose via anaerobic glycolysis to lactic acid. There is a net energy gain by the tumour and net loss by the host result as the host expends energy by converting the lactate back to glucose by the Cori cycle. The alterations in metabolism are suspected, but not yet proven in cats. Hyperlactataemia can result, and this should be taken into consideration if intravenous fluid therapy is required. Hartmann's solution (Lactated Ringer's) can exacerbate any hyperlactataemia and energy demands.

Carbohydrates can be poorly utilised due to peripheral insulin resistance; excess dietary soluble carbohydrates need to be avoided. NFE needs to be ⊆25% of dry matter or ⊆20% of metabolised energy. Providing metabolisable energy from fat is the most beneficial for the animal. Increased dietary fibre may aid in preventing abnormal stool quality (e.g. soft stools or diarrhoea), which is commonly encountered when changing from a high-carbohydrate commercial dry food to a high-fat commercial or homemade diet. Recommendations of crude fibre levels greater than 2.5% DMB are documented [1].

Protein

Tumours use amino acids as a preferred source of energy. This results in an altered metabolism, with the patient having to increase skeletal protein breakdown, liver protein synthesis and whole-body synthesis for tumour growth. This can become clinically significant when protein degradation exceeds intake. The immune response, wound healing rates and gastrointestinal functioning are also affected by the imbalances in protein levels. Specific amino acids have been shown to have different effects in cancer patients.

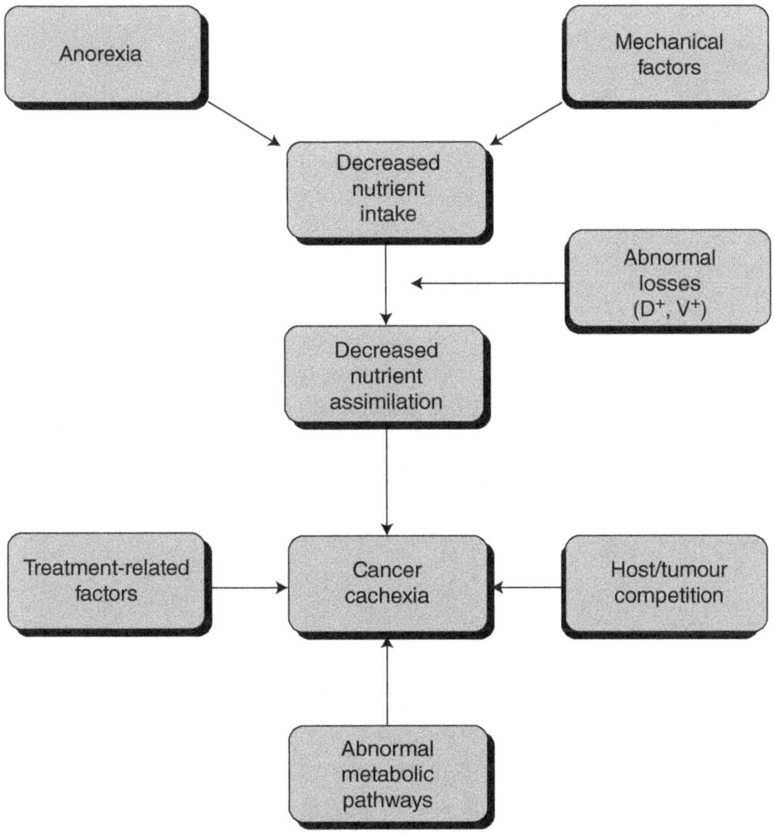

FIGURE 7.1 Diagram demonstrating effects that contribute towards cancer cachexia. D+, diarhhoea; V+, vomiting.

Arginine and glutamine are commonly supplemented in diets specifically designed for cancer patients. The addition of arginine to TPN solutions can decrease tumour growth and metabolic rate in rodent models. In canine models, quality of life and survival time have been increased when fed arginine in conjunction with *n*-3 fatty acids. Glutamine is also added to most human and veterinary enteral formulas. Glutamine is beneficial in improving intestinal morphometry, reducing bacterial translocation, enhancing local immunity and improving survival times. Glutamine is a conditionally essential amino acid. Supplementation is recommended when protein metabolism is altered, as in cancer patients.

The amino acids methionine and asparagine are both used in tumour cell growth. Methionine's precursor, homocysteine, when supplemented in the diet, can stop tumour cell growth progression into different growth phases. This enables cell-cycle-specific therapeutic agents to target more tumour cells. Use of L-asparaginase in dogs and cats with lymphoma has high remission rates of 80%, due to asparagine being an essential factor in cell growth. The supplementation of glycine can also have important implications depending on the type of chemotherapy being utilised. Glycine will reduce cisplatin-induced nephrotoxicity.

Fats

A larger proportion of the metabolisable energy should be from dietary fat and oils. This is due to tumour cells having difficulty utilising fats and oils. If cachexia is present, an increase in dietary fat can improve the body condition scores. 25–40% on a dry matter basis is an ideal dietary fat content, or 50–65% of the calories on an 'as fed basis'. Lipid metabolism also alters in cancer patients. Increased blood concentration of free fatty acids, very low-density lipoproteins, triglycerides, plasma lipoproteins, hormone-dependent lipoproteins and lipase activity can occur due to an overall decrease in lipogenesis and increased lipolysis. These changes in lipid metabolism can also cause immunosuppression, which relates to a decrease in survival time.

Omega-3 (*n*-3) fatty acids, like EPA and DHA, generally have an inhibiting effect on tumour growth. EPA can decrease protein degradation without altering protein synthesis, thus aiding in the symptoms associated with cachexia. The ratio of *n*-3 to *n*-6 fatty acids is important, as omega-6 (*n*-6) fatty acids such as linoleic and γ-linolenic acid enhance metastases.

Vitamins and Minerals

The levels of vitamins and minerals within the diet need to be sufficient to meet daily nutrient intakes. Higher levels of antioxidant vitamins and minerals should be advocated to counteract the damage caused by free radical action and improve immune response. There are two hypotheses surrounding the use of antioxidants in cancer patients. The first supports the role of antioxidants within the diet. They may improve the efficacy of cancer therapy by improving immune function, increasing tumour response to radiation or chemotherapy, decreasing toxicity to normal cells, and helping to reverse metabolic changes contributing towards cachexia [2]. The second hypothesis states that antioxidants may have a deleterious effect by protecting cancer cells against damage by chemotherapy or radiation therapy [2].

Serum levels of the trace minerals zinc, chromium and iron are lower in dogs with lymphoma and osteosarcoma than in healthy dogs [3]. Diets that are complete and balanced should not need supplementation of these trace minerals. Although in homemade diets it should be considered.

FEEDING A CANCER DIET

An initial assessment of the patient needs to be performed. Regular reassessments and calculations of energy requirements will be needed, especially if weight loss or cachexia starts to occur. If hospitalised, patients need to ingest at least their RER.

Due to the discussed altered metabolism processes, modifying nutrient intake is required. Veterinary therapeutic diets are available and, with an increased fat content, are very palatable. A suitable period of transition onto the new diet is required. Some animals, however, can suffer diarrhoea due to the increase in fat content and may need a longer period of transition.

With all cancer patients, care should be taken with monitoring weight loss, especially with those who are initially overweight. Rapid weight loss, due to anorexia and alterations in metabolism, can result in a loss of lean muscle mass. Fat stores may remain and may mask the detrimental effect of protein catabolism. Careful muscle condition scores and body condition scores will need to be performed, as 'overcoat syndrome' can quite easily be present.

The use of appetite stimulants can be useful in some cancer patients, with mirtazapine being the most common. If appetite stimulants fail and long-term nutritional support is required, enteral feeding techniques do need to be considered. Active encouragement to eat still needs to be initiated by the owner or practice staff if hospitalised. If the animal is nauseous due to illness or medication, refer back to the veterinary surgeon, as controlling the nausea is vital in encouraging calorie intake.

Support for the owner is greatly required with cancer patients. The word cancer will make any owner anxious, especially if the animal is anorexic, which can be very distressing. Many animals will be susceptible to this in their owners, and it can be another factor associated with anorexia.

REFERENCES

1. Sheng-Long, Y.E., Istafan, N.W., and Driscoll, D.F. (1992). Tumour and host response to arginine and branch chain amino acid enriched total parenteral nutrition. *Cancer* 69: 261–270.
2. Roudebush, P., Davenport, D.J., and Novotny, B.J. (2004). The use of nutraceuticals in cancer therapy. *Vet. Clin. Small Anim.* 34: 249–269.
3. Kazmierski, K.J., Ogilvie, G.K., Fettman, M.J. et al. (2001). Serum zinc, chromium and iron concentrations in dogs with lymphoma and osteosarcoma. *J. Vet. Intern. Med.* 15: 585–588.

CHAPTER 8

Cardiac Disease

The aims of clinical nutrition are:

- To help control signs associated with sodium and fluid retention by avoiding nutritional deficiencies and excesses
- To aid in maintaining normal heart muscle function
- To slow the progression of possible concurrent renal disease
- To support patients receiving diuretics or angiotensin-converting enzyme (ACE) inhibitors/blockers
- To maintain optimum body condition score and lean muscle mass, aiding in the prevention of cardiac cachexia

The nutritional status of the cardiac patient is exceptionally important to ascertain as this can have several effects on the patient. This can include the choice and dose rate of the drugs used in the medical treatment, interpretation of any laboratory results, interpretation of ECG data, prognosis of both surgical and medical intervention and the choice of diet for the patient. As part of the initial clinical assessment, a full history of the animal's diet should be taken. Nutrition can be a causative factor in cardiac disease. If the animal receives unusual supplements, is not fed a complete diet, if more than one animal in the household is affected, or if it is being fed a homemade or fad diet, cardiac disease can be induced. Micro- and macronutrient deficiencies can cause cardiac problems, and thus, a complete blood workup needs to be performed.

Assessment of body condition and muscle scores of each animal is important in cardiac patients. A reduction in skeletal muscle mass might indicate energy malnutrition and possibly a negative nitrogen balance. Animals with catabolic disease, such as hyperthyroidism in cats and cardiac failure, lose body mass very rapidly, as with anorexic cats. The progression of cardiac disease can be exacerbated in obese animals. This can result in cardiomegaly, circulatory congestion, oedema, ascites and hypocalcaemia. An overweight animal must be subjectively assessed; obesity must be differentiated from abdominal distension due to hepatomegaly or ascites. Obesity can

Box 8.1 Cardiovascular adaptations that occur during the transition from ideal body score to obesity

- Increased perfusion requirements of expanding adipose tissue
- Elevated cardiac output
- Abnormal left ventricular function
- Variable blood pressure response (normotensive to hypertensive)
- Increased retention of sodium and water by the kidney
- Increased plasma aldosterone and norepinephrine (noradrenaline) concentration
- Increased left arterial pressure
- Increased heart rate
- Exercise intolerance

also mask an underlying lean muscle mass. Obesity not only produces clinical signs (Box 8.1) that mimic those of early heart failure, but it can also cause cardiovascular changes that can exacerbate any underlying cardiovascular disease.

CARDIAC CACHEXIA

Notably, 34–75% of dogs suffering from heart disease suffer from anorexia, and it is one of the multifactorial processes associated with the loss of lean body mass in cardiac cachexia [1]. Other factors include increased energy requirements and metabolic alterations. Cardiac cachexia is more commonly seen in dogs than in cats and in DCM or right-sided heart failure. The primary energy source for animals with acute or chronic disease is amino acids from muscle, thus causing a reduction in lean body mass. Cachexia is a slow, progressive process of the loss of lean body mass/muscle. Careful examinations of obese animals should occur, as this lean body mass reduction can occur, creating overcoat syndrome, and be easily missed. Any clinical nutrition of these animals includes the management of any anorexia that is present.

CLINICAL NUTRITION

L-Carnitine

L-Carnitine is critical for fatty acid metabolism and energy production, and cardiac myocytes depend upon the oxidation of fatty acids for their energy. L-Carnitine deficiencies and a causative link with DCM have not been established. L-Carnitine deficiencies within the cardiac myocytes occur in 50% of dogs suffering from DCM. Some affected dogs with DCM do respond to L-carnitine supplementation. Carnitine supplementation of 50–100 mg/kg bwt orally every eight hours has been recommended to dogs with DCM [1], though most cardiac diets are already supplemented with L-carnitine.

Fats

The role of fatty acids in the diet of cardiac patients has been widely reported. Supplementation of the diet with EPA and DHA has been shown to improve cachexia scores but has no effect on survival time, thus improving quality of life. Animals suffering from cardiac cachexia have increased production of inflammatory cytokines. These cytokines are directly linked to causing anorexia, to increasing energy requirements and to increasing catabolism of lean body mass [1]. Supplementation of the diet with omega-3 fatty acids (especially EPA and DHA) decreases the production and effects of cytokines.

Recommended dosage of 40 mg/kg bwt of EPA and 25 mg/kg bwt of DHA for both dogs and cats with anorexia or cachexia has been noted [1]. With most fish oil supplements containing 180 mg EPA and 120 mg of DHA per capsule, dosages can be easily calculated [1]. Specific fatty acid supplements are now available for cardiac patients.

Medium chain triglycerides (MCTs) have been shown to have a large positive effect on mitochondrial function in the cardiomyocytes. MCTs do not require carnitine-mediated transport to cross the mitochondrial membrane. They are, therefore, readily available as an energy source in the cardiomyocytes.

Carbohydrates

The level of carbohydrates in the diet has to support adequate calories for the specific life stage. The recommended fibre levels in the diet are very much dependent on the individual. If the animal is obese, it is initially recommended that the animal reduce in weight and reach it's optimal body weight and BCS. This may involve the use of a high-fibre diet. In animals, which are already at an ideal BCS and optimal weight, fibre should be present but not excessive. The presence of fibre in the diet does reduce the bioavailability of many of the nutrients. As concurrent disease or impairment of the gastrointestinal tract, pancreas and liver may occur, a high-fibre diet is not ideal [2].

Vitamins and Minerals

The nutrients of main concern in patients with heart failure include sodium, potassium and magnesium. Treats and snacks, which are often fed to dogs, do have a high salt content, as do cheese and processed meats, which are often used to administer medications. The restriction of sodium in the diet is useful in the mechanism to reduce fluid retention that accompanies many forms of heart disease. Both sodium and water can be retained when the renin–angiotensin–aldosterone (RAA) cascade is stimulated or when the patient's blood pressure falls [3]. One of the current methods of treatment for fluid retention is the use of diuretics. The diuretics block sodium retention but also promote urinary loss of magnesium and potassium. The prolonged use of diuretics can also lead to deficiencies of the water-soluble vitamins.

As a result of the cascade being stimulated, extracellular and vascular fluid volume increases, thus increasing preload. The plasma protein concentration, therefore, becomes more dilute, which in turn decreases plasma oncotic pressure. Water moves from the vascular to the interstitial compartment, resulting in oedema, ascites and congestion.

The use of ACE inhibitors has led to modification of the recommendation for sodium restriction, from senior diets and early cardiac disease diets. ACE inhibitors are designed to block the production of angiotensin II and its subsequent stimulation of the secretion of aldosterone. Both of these chemicals promote the retention of water and sodium by the kidneys. Thus, ACE inhibitors result in impaired sodium and water excretion. Sodium intake needs to be limited in proportion to the severity of the disease (see Table 8.1), in an attempt to avoid excesses. ACE inhibitors can also cause the retention of potassium; thus, periodic serum levels should be monitored [4]. Spironolactone has similar potassium-sparing effects, along with being an aldosterone antagonist. CRF is often a concomitant disease of patients with cardiovascular disorders. Diets for these animals also need restricted phosphorus levels. Levels of potassium and magnesium should also be optimally controlled, as they support the patient receiving diuretics and/or ACE inhibitor therapy.

Magnesium levels can have a deleterious effect on a range of cardiovascular conditions, including hypertension, congestive heart failure, coronary artery disease and cardiac arrhythmias [4]. Hypomagnesaemia can be induced through the use of digoxin and loop diuretics.

The B vitamin complexes are often supplemented in cardiac diets. At present, there has been little investigation into the role of vitamin B deficiency as a cause of heart disease in dogs and cats. Polyuria and anorexia can both contribute to low vitamin B concentrations, and thus, higher B vitamin requirements are needed.

TABLE 8.1 Nutrition guidelines for MMVD.

Stage A No formal recommendation	• Feed a complete and balanced diet that supports an ideal body condition score
Stage B1 No formal recommendation	• Feed a complete and balanced diet that supports an ideal body condition score
Stage B2 Mild sodium restriction (<100 mg/100 kcal)	• Feed a complete and balanced diet • Provide adequate calories and protein for optimal body condition • Determine what type of palatability enhancers the patient might enjoy

Stage C/D
Modest sodium restriction
(<75 mg/100 kcal)
	• Feed a complete and balanced diet
	• Feed a highly palatable diet
	• Prevent cachexia
	  • Maintain adequate calories and protein
	  • Consider omega-3 fatty acids
	  • Monitor for nutrient excess and deficiencies

Adapted from Ref. [5].

Recommendations of higher levels of antioxidants in animals suffering from CHF are commonplace due to the by-products of ROS. Coenzyme Q_{10}, another antioxidant, has also been anecdotally recommended. Coenzyme Q_{10}, like carnitine, is a cofactor in several energy-producing reactions. Benefits of supplementation include improved myocardial metabolic efficiency and increases in antioxidant production [1]. Although no direct evidence has been achieved in establishing Coenzyme Q_{10}'s direct benefits, recommended dosages of 30 mg orally bid and, in large breed dogs, up to 90 mg bid PO have been reported [1].

Proteins

Taurine is an essential amino acid in cats due to taurine being the only amino acid able to combine with cholesterol during bile salt synthesis, whereas in other species, another amino acid, glycine, can be substituted. Cats do have a limited ability to synthesise taurine from cysteine and methionine, but its use outstrips production. The mechanism of heart failure in cats and dogs with taurine deficiency is poorly understood. Prior to 1987, supplementation of commercial foods with taurine was not commonplace, and the number of cases of feline DCM was large. Clinical studies have also shown that inadequate potassium intake may be sufficient to induce a significant taurine depletion and cardiovascular disease in cats. Most dogs presenting with DCM do not tend to have a concurrent taurine deficiency. Although in some breeds, where DCM is not a common disease, a taurine deficiency has been noted. Dog breeds reported to be associated with taurine deficiency include the American cocker spaniel, golden retriever, Labrador, Newfoundland, Dalmatian and English bulldog [1].

The overall protein level in the diet is reduced. This is due to the progression of renal disease, which is associated with cardiac disease. The protein levels are therefore restricted, but of a high biological value; typical values of 17% (DMB) for dogs and 29% (DMB) for cats are often recommended. This can equate to 5.5 g/100 kcal to help maintain lean body mass.

It should be noted that if protein restriction is too restricted, this can be detrimental to the animal. Protein malnutrition can rapidly occur in the presence of catabolic disease and inadequate food intake. Hypoproteinaemia can be present in cardiac disease with reduced liver function.

FEEDING THE CARDIAC PATIENT

Each diet must be based on each individual's specific requirements. Overweight or obese animals will require diets aimed at calorie-restricted diets, whilst underweight patients will require a calorie-dense diet. Concurrent disease also needs to be taken into consideration. Laboratory parameters should be obtained to identify any electrolyte excesses or deficiencies. Anorexia is a common side effect of CHF, and great effort on behalf of the owner may be required in order to entice the animal to eat (Table 8.1).

FEEDING A LOW-SALT DIET

Low-salt diets are used for both cardiac and renal patients. It is often a misconception that low-salt diets have reduced palatability. Studies have demonstrated that diets with reduced sodium chloride levels used in patients with cardiovascular or renal disease have comparable or better palatability than supermarket brands [6]. Difficulties in transition from the patient's original diet to a low-salt prescription diet can be attributed to:

1. Advanced illness associated with renal and heart failure.
2. Established eating and feeding habits of both the animal and the owner.
3. Anorexia is associated with the disease process and/or medications.
4. Too quick a transition and/or established food aversions.

Transition to a low-salt diet is always easier if the animal has already been fed a diet in a lower salt category. Animals are often encouraged to consume a new diet by adding flavour enhancers. Low-sodium additives can include low-sodium soups and sweeteners, such as honey or syrups. As with all clinical prescription diets, the therapeutic agent of the diet should not be imposed if it is detrimental to the overall nutrient intake. Owners should be aware that both trial and error might be required in these patients. Some animals can 'go off' certain diets, and a cyclical approach with two or three commercial prescription diets may be required. Use of different feeding methods along with different foods should be utilised. The success of a transition to a new diet hugely depends on the dedication of the owner and the support received by the veterinary practice. Supporting the owner can be achieved by providing a list of foodstuffs and their sodium content.

Administering medications can be difficult, and many of the foods used to 'hide' medications can be high in salt. Advising owners on different methods can aid in an increase in compliance. Alternatives can include:

- Teaching the owner to administer medications without the use of food. This can include the use of pill givers.
- The use of commercial treats designed to hold medications. Always double-check the salt content.
- Use of appropriate foods such as bananas (good potassium source), no-added-salt peanut butter (not ideal in obese animals) and home-cooked meats (without added salt), not sandwich/processed meats.

REFERENCES

1. Freeman, L.M. and Rush, J.E. (2017). Nutritional modulation of heart disease Chapter 177. In: *Textbook of Veterinary Internal Medicine*, 8e, vol. 1 (ed. S.J. Ettinger and E.C. Feldman), 1800–1805.
2. Roudebush, P. Study cited in Roudebush, P., Keene, B.W., and Mizelle, L.(2000). Cardiovascular disease. In: *Small Animal Clinical Nutrition*, 4e (ed. M.S. Hand, C.D. Thatcher, R.L. Remillard, and P. Roudebush), 529–562. Missouri: Mark Morris Institute.

3. Davies, M. (1996). Feeding the cardiac patient. In: *BSAVA Manual of Companion Animal Nutrition and Feeding* (ed. N. Kelly and J. Wills), 117–127. Gloucester: BSAVA Publications.
4. Buffington, T., Holloway, C., and Abood, S. (2004). *Manual of Veterinary Dietetics.* Missouri: Elsevier Saunders.
5. Torres, C. (2023). Cardiac disease in dogs. In: *Purina Institute Handout of Canine and Feline Clinical Nutrition*. St. Louis, MO: Purina Institute.
6. Roudebush, P., Keene, B.W., and Mizelle, L. (2000). Cardiovascular disease. In: *Small Animal Clinical Nutrition*, 4e (ed. M.S. Hand, C.D. Thatcher, R.L. Remillard, and P. Roudebush), 529–562. Missouri: Mark Morris Institute.

CHAPTER 9

Supportive Feeding Methods in Small Animals

SUMMARY

The use of feeding tubes in the delivery of nutrition (calories and nutrients) is an important aspect to consider as part of the nutritional assessment. Consideration should be given to the calorific value required, the diet to be used (including what diets are available), the form in which the diet is to be delivered, whether the animal is able to consume, digest and absorb the diet and the composition of the nutrients within the diet.

INTRODUCTION

With all sick companion animals, the nutritional goal is for the patient to eat the designated diet in sufficient quantities. Critically sick animals in a hospital environment, where the added stress of this different environment can affect food consumption and metabolism. Many animals may require, or benefit from, a veterinary therapeutic diet, but the initial goal is to ensure that the patient is receiving their daily calorific requirement from a nutritionally balanced diet. Analgesia should not be forgotten, as pain can reduce food intake in some animals, as can nausea. Pharmaceutical intervention can also be utilised to aid with nausea. Hydration and electrolyte status must be maintained and corrected before any nutritional support can be initiated. The aim of critical care nutrition is dependent on the disease process and/or the individual's specific requirements. Each case must be considered on its specific requirements once a full clinical examination and history (including nutritional history) have been achieved [1]. The sole aim can be defined as to prevent and/or treat malnutrition when present. To define any nutritional aims in more depth, it is more beneficial to split the aims into short-term and long-term goals.

The short-term aims are to:

- Provide for any ongoing nutritional requirements (both in terms of energy and nutrients).
- Prevent or correct any nutritional deficiencies or imbalances.
- Minimise metabolic derangements.
- Prevention of further catabolism of lean body mass.

Long-term nutritional aims should include:

- Restoration of optimal body condition (optimum body condition score (BCS) and muscle condition score (MCS)).
- Provide required nutrients to the animal within its own environment.

As disease processes change and the animal's physiological and metabolic responses alter the nature of the nutritional support, both the short-term and long-term nutritional aims may alter.

When assessing animals for the preferred method of critical care feeding, the nutritional status of the animal needs to be evaluated. This should include BCS, MCS, hydration status, weight, hair coat quality, signs of inadequate wound healing, hypoalbuminemia, lymphopenia and coagulopathy [2]. Thought should be given to 'fluid shifts' in these animals as they can severely affect haematological values and the animal's weight. Factors that should be identified include specific electrolyte imbalances, hyperglycaemia, hypertriglyceridemia or hyperammonaemia, as they will have large consequences on the nutritional critical care plan [3]. Adequate adjustments will be required to the feeding plan.

CLINICAL NUTRITION

Water (Hydration Levels)

The initial stage of nutritional support is correcting any dehydration, electrolyte replacement and normalisation of the acid-base status before starting assisted feeding. Initiating assisted feeding before the patient is haemodynamically stable can further compromise the patient. If oedema occurs or dehydration persists, recalculation of flow rates is required. Monitoring of hydration level indicators is required during intravenous fluid therapy. Daily maintenance fluid requirements are approximately 50–60 ml/kg bwt/day, or 2 ml/kg bwt/hour. If persistent vomiting or diarrhoea is present, these additional losses need to be factored in. Urine output should also be monitored. For every 1% dehydration, there is a fluid deficit of 10 ml/kg. This deficit should then be replaced over a 24–48-hour period.

Percentage of dehydration	**Clinical signs**
<5%	No obvious outward signs Concentrated urine
5–8%	Slightly prolonged CRT Slight tenting of the skin Mucous membranes feel tacky Third eyelid visible
8–10%	Sunken eyes Prolonged CRT Obvious tenting of the skin
10–12%	Oliguria Tented skin remains in place Clinical shock can be experienced
>12%	Progressive shock Coma and death.

10 kg dog with 10% dehydration needs 50–60 ml/kg bwt/day plus the deficit. Daily fluid requirement is 500–600 ml/day; the deficit (10%) is at 10 ml/kg for each 1% = 1,000 ml.

Protein

Protein energy malnutrition (PEM) can occur during periods of illness, injury or even after routine operations. During these periods, the body shuts down systems to conserve the limited resources. Physiological changes such as a drop in blood pressure, reduction in cardiac output and a drop in oxygen consumption occur. This is clinical shock and is known as the Ebb phase. Clinical shock is treatable, but the length of time that shock is suffered from is variable and can ultimately be lethal. Following the Ebb phase is the flow or hypermetabolic phase. During this second phase, the patient's body defence and repair mechanisms are initiated. This process is where anorexia and starvation differ [4].

Patients in a catabolic state will utilise the skeletal muscle proteins; nutritional support with adequate protein levels for the specific life stage and nutritional assessment is vital. Sufficient calories need to be supplied to the patient from fats and carbohydrates. This will ensure that proteins are not used as a source of energy. The quality of the proteins provided is of importance, as is the digestibility. Specific amino acids are supplemented to commercially available critical care diets. Glutamine is an important substrate for the increased levels of gluconeogenesis, used in rapidly dividing cells. Any deficiency in this amino acid has been shown to lead to gut mucosal atrophy and an increase in bacterial translocation due to a compromise of the mucosal barrier. This can lead to the suggestion that glutamine may behave as a 'conditionally essential' amino acid during severe illness. The essential amino acid arginine has a positive effect on the immune system and can subsequently improve survival times of septic patients. Many enteral diets are supplemented with both glutamine and arginine. High doses of glutamine have a trophic effect on the gut mucosa.

The use of a novel protein source in these cases has been advocated. It has been postulated that an intestinal inflammatory environment can play a role in the formation of food allergies [5]. This has also been hypothesised in cases of inflammatory bowel disease (IBD) [6].

Vitamins and Minerals

The supplementation of vitamins and minerals for hospitalised patients will depend on the disease and the severity of that disease that is present. Sodium, chloride, potassium, phosphate, calcium and magnesium should be used for short-term nutritional support. All animals that receive intravenous fluid therapy with or without parenteral support should have daily electrolyte levels monitored. If any polydipsia or polyuria is present, supplementation of the water-soluble vitamins is required [7]. Zinc aids in promoting wound healing and plays a role in protein and nucleic acid metabolism. Supplementation of nutritional support diets with zinc has been recommended.

Carbohydrates

Carbohydrates within any critical care diet need to be of a very high digestibility. The quantities of fibre need to be kept to a minimum, as this will decrease digestibility and bind up important nutrients. The crude fibre concentrations are generally very low at 3–6.9 g/1,000 kcal and 1.2 g/1,000 kcal in 'recovery diets' and liquid diets, respectively [8]. The level of carbohydrate in the diet needs to be adequate to supply the required calories for recovery.

Fats

The quantity of fat in a critical care diet does need to be increased. A higher level of calories can be obtained from fat rather than from carbohydrates. The inclusion of omega-3 fatty acids can help decrease any inflammatory response. Liquid and recovery diets will contain, on average, 45–47% and 55–68% calories from fat, respectively [8].

SUPPORTIVE FEEDING METHODS

Supportive feeding methods should be considered when there is a history of greater than 10% weight loss, decreased food intake, anorexia, increased nutrient demands due to trauma or surgery, increased nutrient losses resulting from vomiting, diarrhoea, burns or scalds, and acute exacerbation of chronic disease. Also, if specific areas of the alimentary canal need to be bypassed (Figure 9.1). The ideal diet to use in these cases should be highly palatable, digestible and have a high energy density. A relatively

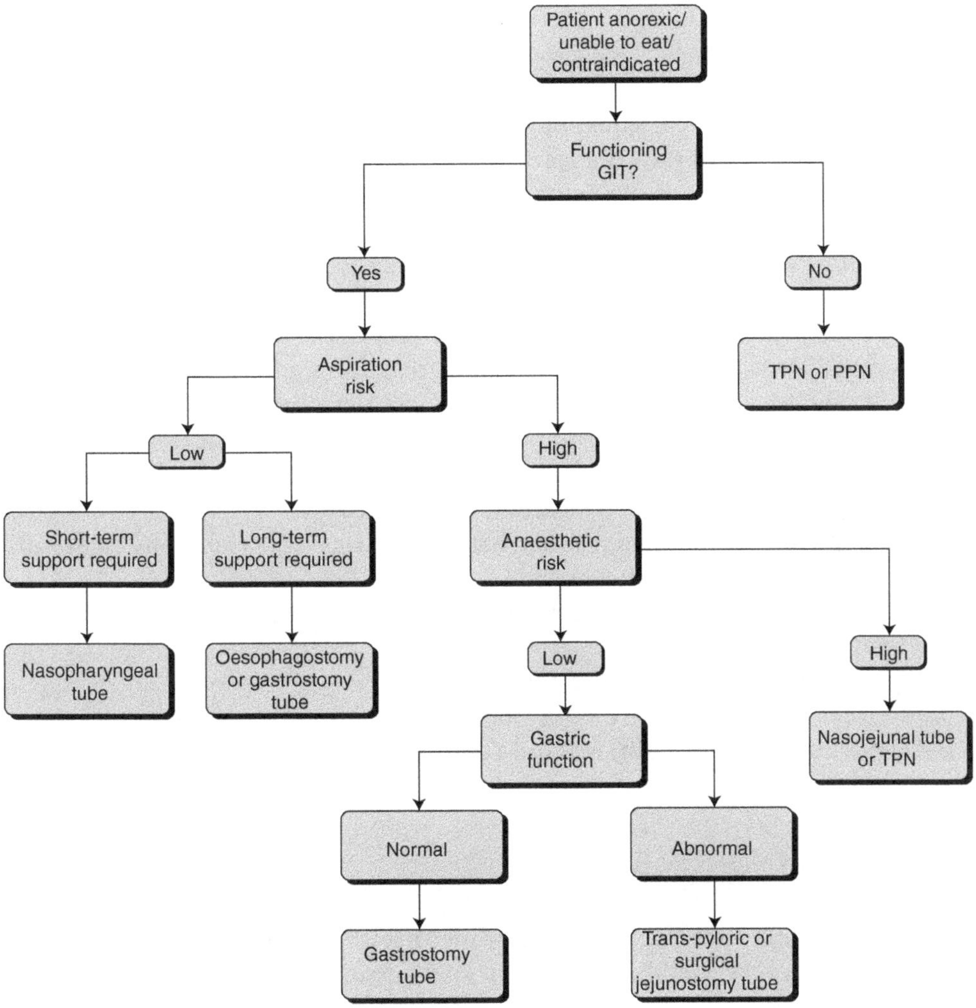

FIGURE 9.1 Flow diagram of assisted feeding decisions.

high percentage of energy should be achieved from protein and fat rather than carbohydrates. The percentage of total calories from digestible carbohydrates in the liquid enteral diets is typically restricted to 21–25% [8].

Critical care diets for cats and dogs are available in three different forms: powdered, liquid and moist diets. Moist diets can have thixotrophic consistencies; when mixed, their viscosity decreases, becoming thinner.

The use of assisted feeding methods does have great advantages, but care of the feeding tube is vital. The artificial opening into the gastrointestinal tract (GIT) through which the tube (O-tube or G-tube) is inserted is referred to as a stoma. The stoma must be treated as a surgical wound and cleaned daily with normal saline or cooled boiled water for the first seven to 14 days, or until it is healed. Dressings around tubes are not always necessary, unless indicated, for example, if the stoma site is infected or the animal is interfering with the insertion site. The tube should always be checked to ensure that it is still situated within the GIT before administration of any diets. This can be achieved by slow administration of water into the tube, assessing for any coughing or sneezing. Radiography can also aid in assessing the location of the tube, but it can't be achieved at every feeding. Use of a capnograph can be utilised. If a trace, similar to an anesthetised patient, is seen, then it implies the tube has moved into the trachea. This is a potential, especially with naso-oesophageal feeding tubes.

The volume of liquid diets administered at each bolus feeding in dogs and cats should not exceed 10–12 ml/kg of body weight (including tube flush volumes) [9]. This is only an estimate, and each animal should be judged on an individual basis. Tolerance to liquid diets is best when small feedings are delivered frequently. Some animals will benefit from trickle feeding; a syringe driver can be utilised to instigate a constant-rate infusion of the diet.

Also, need to be very careful not to overperfuse any animals that are also being tube fed. Most diets are 80% water (without extra added).

If you tube feed the animal 4 times a day with 5 ml before and after = 40 ml of water in total per day as a flush.

3 kg DSH needs 140 ml of a diet (at 80% moisture), which would be = 112 ml of fluid per day.

Daily total of 152 ml going down the tube.

Daily fluid requirements are 50–60 ml/kg/day = 150–180 ml needed per day for our 3 kg DSH example. No additional fluid requirements are needed.

REFEEDING SYNDROME

Refeeding syndrome (RFS) is a potentially life-threatening metabolic condition that occurs when a severely malnourished or starved animal is reintroduced to food too quickly.

THE PATHOPHYSIOLOGY

The syndrome is driven by a massive shift in how the body processes energy (Figure 9.2):

- Starvation State: During long-term fasting, the body switches from burning carbohydrates to burning its own fat and muscle. Intracellular stores of electrolytes – phosphorus, potassium and magnesium – become severely depleted, though blood levels often appear deceptively normal.
- The Refeeding Trigger: When food (especially carbohydrates) is reintroduced, the pancreas releases a large burst of insulin to process the new glucose.
- The Metabolic Crash: This insulin surge forces the already low electrolytes to rush out of the blood and into the cells to assist with metabolism. This causes the blood levels of these minerals to plummet dangerously low.

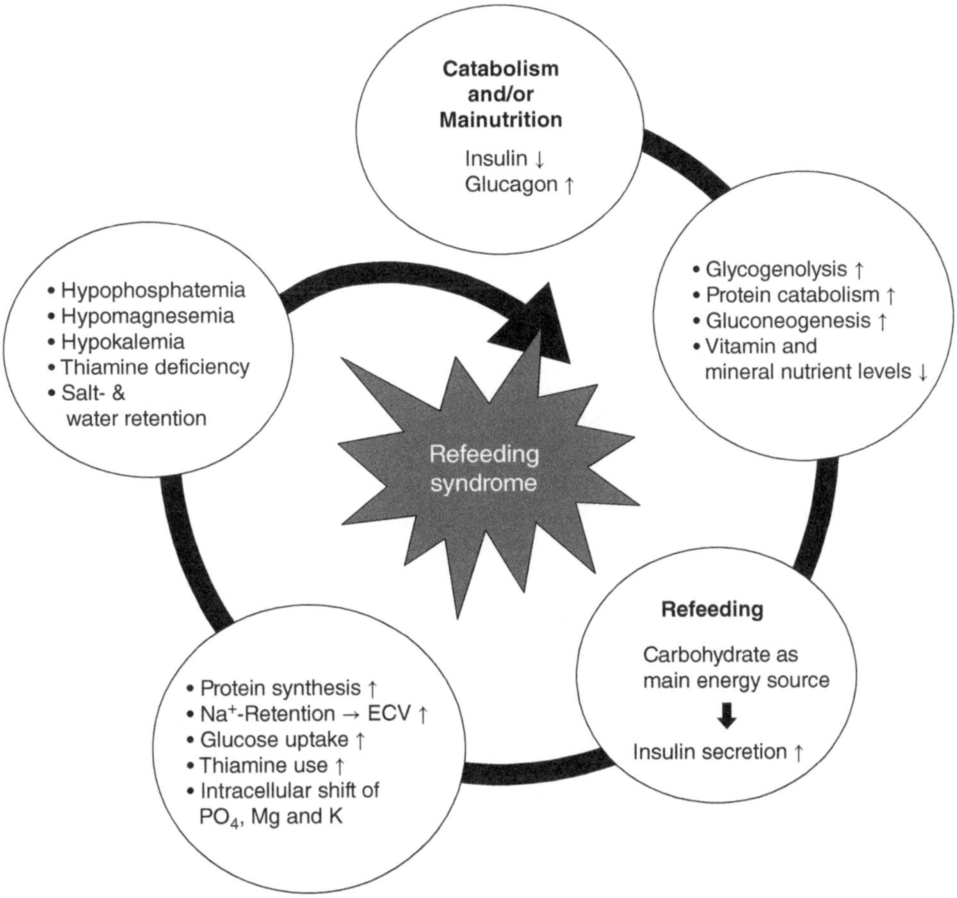

FIGURE 9.2 Pathophysiology of refeeding syndrome. Adapted from [1].

CRITICAL MINERAL DEFICIENCIES

- Hypophosphatemia: The 'hallmark' of RFS. It can cause red blood cell breakdown (haemolysis), heart failure and respiratory muscle paralysis.
- Hypokalaemia: Leads to life-threatening heart arrhythmias and extreme muscle weakness.
- Hypomagnesaemia: Causes tremors, seizures, and can make potassium deficiencies impossible to correct.
- Thiamine (Vitamin B1) Deficiency: Carbohydrate metabolism rapidly consumes the body's remaining thiamine, potentially causing severe neurological symptoms.

If not managed, these shifts lead to multisystem organ failure, including cardiac arrest, pulmonary oedema and seizures.

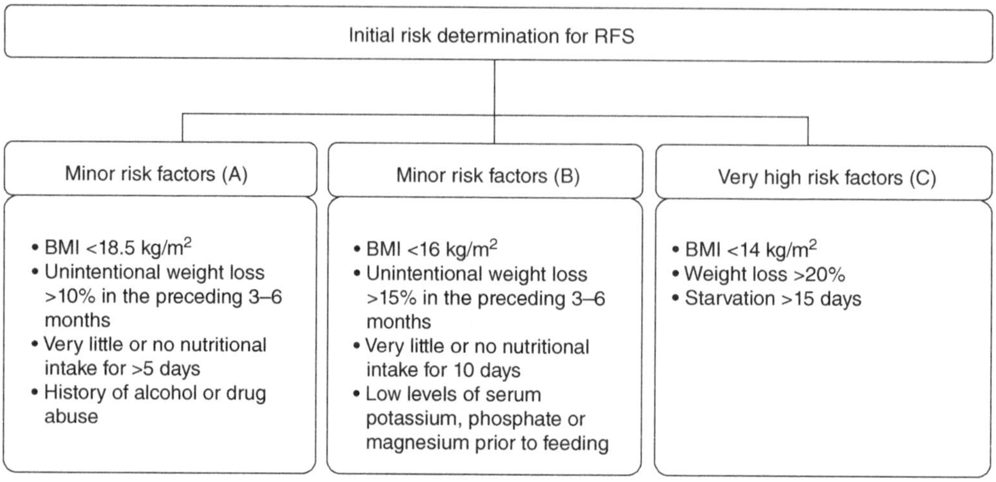

FIGURE 9.3 Protocol used in human medicine to determine risk factors for RFS. Ref. [9] / with permission of John Wiley & Sons.

When assessing animals for the preferred method of critical care feeding, the nutritional status of the animal needs to be evaluated. This should include BCS, MCS, hydration status, weight, hair coat quality, signs of inadequate wound healing, hypoalbuminemia, lymphopenia and coagulopathy [2]. Thought should be given to 'fluid shifts' in these animals as they can severely affect haematological values and the animal's weight. Factors that should be identified include specific electrolyte imbalances, hyperglycaemia, hypertriglyceridemia or hyperammonaemia, as they will have large consequences on the nutritional critical care plan [3]. Adequate adjustments will be required to the feeding plan.

The goal is to reintroduce calories slowly to prevent RFS. The mechanisms that lead to RFS will occur in all animals (that can produce insulin); it's the magnitude of this insulin surge and the knock-on effect of the electrolyte disturbances that will differ. In human medicine, the treatment regimen will depend on the baseline electrolyte levels and risk factors of the patient (Figure 9.3). Many of the risk factors are not relevant to veterinary medicine but do highlight that some of these elements can be applied, for example length of inappetence/starvation and BCS, rather than BMI.

1. Baseline levels of phosphorus, potassium and magnesium.
2. Begin at 25% of the animal's resting energy requirement (RER) for the first 24 hours, with close monitoring of electrolytes.
3. Divide the daily allowance into 4–6 small meals.
4. Use a high-fat, low-carbohydrate and high-protein diet to minimise insulin spikes. Avoid diets that are restricted in any of the electrolytes, including phosphates.
5. Increase by 1/8 to 1/4 of the total requirement every one to two days until reaching full RER. Traditionally, this was stated as three days, increasing by a third each day. A more personalised approach should be taken, dependent on electrolyte and glucose levels (see Figure 9.4).
6. Supplementation: Thiamine (Vitamin B1) and electrolytes as required [10, 11].

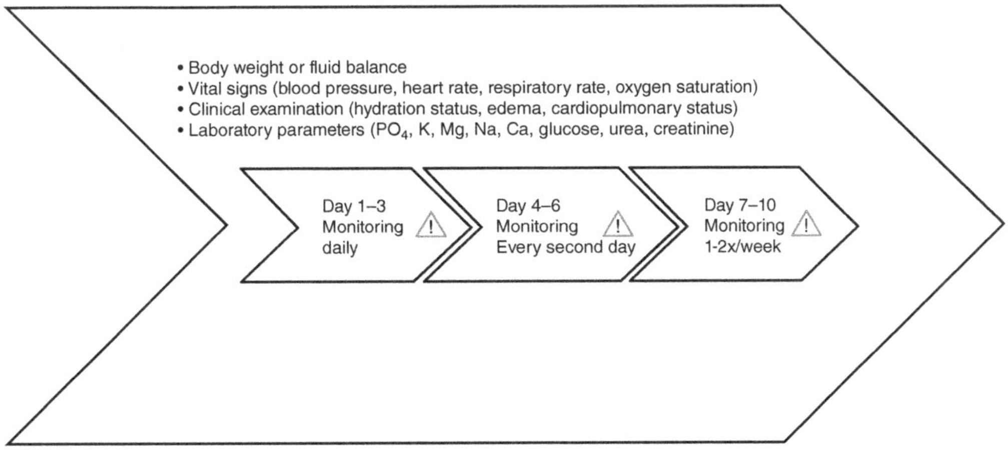

FIGURE 9.4 Monitoring schematic for RFS. Ref. [9] / with permission of John Wiley & Sons.

Encouraging Animals to Eat

The process of encouraging animals to eat should never be forgotten. Voluntary intake can be established in some cases by taking time out to personally encourage the animal to eat. Grooming can actively encourage the animals (especially dogs and cats) to eat, removing a nasal discharge that is blocking their sense of smell, as can TLC, providing competition, hand feeding, providing a selection of different diets, and if possible, taking the animal into a different environment.

Microenteral Nutrition

Microenteral nutrition is the delivery of very small amounts of water, electrolytes, and easily absorbable nutrients directly into the GIT. This method is often underused in veterinary practices, but it allows for the nutritional requirements of the intestinal mucosa. This helps to preserve the intestinal blood flow, the mucosal barrier, and its immune function [12]. Initial volumes of 0.05 to 0.2 ml/kg bwt/hour are recommended and will add exceptionally little to the volume of fluids normally produced by the stomach. Gradual increases can occur to 1–2 ml/kg bwt/hour over a 24 to 48-hour period. Enteral solutions that can be used include oral rehydrating solutions and those containing glutamine. This method of nutrient delivery can be administered orally or via feeding tubes.

Naso-Oesophageal/Gastric Tubes

Naso tubes (Figure 9.5) are generally well tolerated by cats and dogs and are suitable for short-term nutritional support, usually three to seven days, though longer periods have been documented. Contraindications for the use of these tubes include unconsciousness, vomiting, disease or dysfunction of the pharynx, larynx, nares, swallowing reflex, oesophagus and stomach. The preferred end placement of the naso tube is debated, whether the tube ends in the caudal oesophagus or the stomach. There is no direct evidence to support either placement.

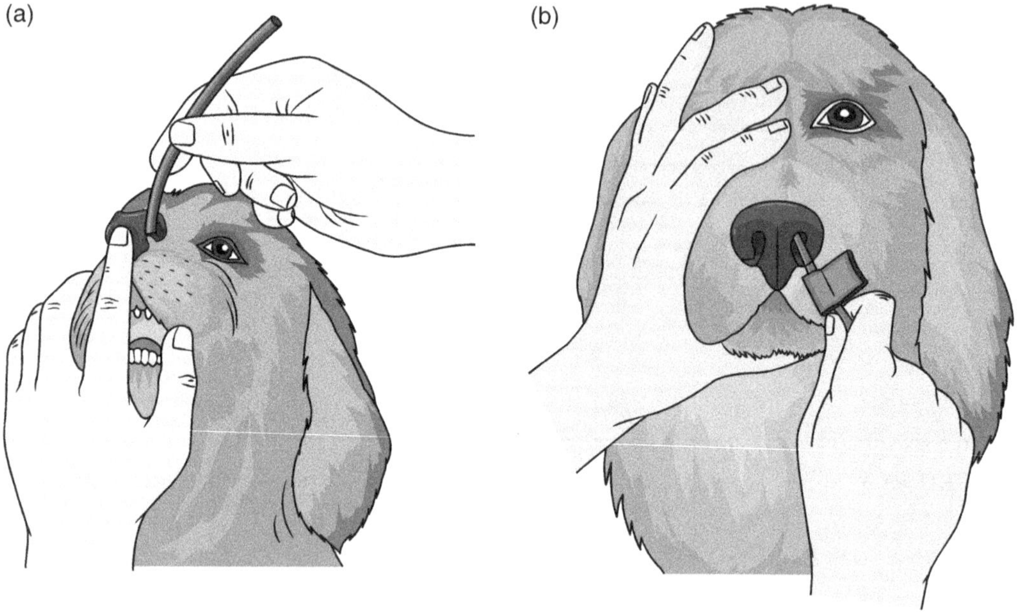

FIGURE 9.5 Placement of a naso-oesphageal tube. (a) Placement of local anaesthetic into the nose is required. After the required period of time for the anaesthetic to work, the external nares are pushed dorsally and the tube is gently passed into the ventral nasal meatus. (b) The tube is fully inserted until the pen mark or adhesive tape tabs are reached. Glue or sutures are then used to secure the tube in position. It is, however, useful to check correct placement of the tube prior to securing.

Once the tube has been placed, a small amount of water is administered slowly into the tube to see if a cough reflex is induced, indicating aspiration. Lateral radiographs can also identify that the tube has been correctly placed. Due to the narrow bore of the tube, blockages can occur. Administration of 5–10 ml of water into the tube post-administration of the liquid diet should aid in the prevention of any blockages. If blockages do occur, small amounts of carbonated drinks, cranberry juice or solutions of pancreatic enzymes have been shown to aid in their removal. Pre-feeding administration of water is required to ensure that the tube is still positioned correctly. Attaching a capnograph to the tube can also help to establish the location of the feeding tube, oesophagus or trachea. Post-water flush is also required to prevent blockages.

Oesophagostomy Tubes

Oesophagostomy tubes (Figure 9.6) are commonly used in cats that have suffered facial trauma. These tubes are of use when bypassing the nose and mouth is required to administer nutritional support. Animals that don't tolerate naso-oesophageal tubes well can have oesophagostomy tubes placed. Aseptic placement of the tube under general anaesthetic is required. Frequent cleaning and inspection of the tube is necessary

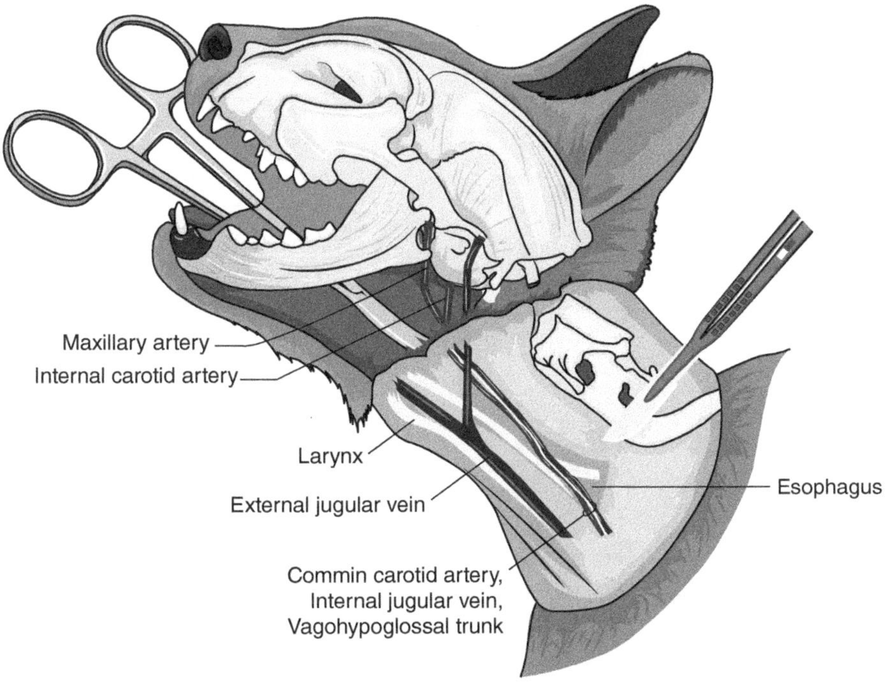

FIGURE 9.6 Placement of an oesphageal feeding tube in a cat.

under aseptic conditions. Complications can include airway obstruction, damage to the cervical nerves and blood vessels, and infections.

Percutaneous Endoscopic Gastrostomy (PEG) Tubes

Placement of these tubes (Figure 9.7) is required under general anaesthesia and needs to be in place for at least five days before removal. PEG tubes are utilised when long-term nutritional support is required and when oesophageal problems are present (e.g. megaoesophagus). Adhesions between the gastric serosa and the peritoneum can form within 48–72 hours. It should be noted that in malnourished patients, these adhesions might take longer to form. Once the tube is placed, only a third of the calculated daily energy requirements should be administered on day two, two-thirds on day three, and by the third day, the full amount. If feedings or volume are not well tolerated, small, more frequent meals can be administered. In some cases, using a syringe driver to maintain a trickle feed can be advantageous. Feeding through the PEG tube can commence four hours after its insertion. If patients are unable to take fluids orally, mouth care should be encouraged at least every four hours. This involves ensuring that the mucous membranes remain moist and that bacterial infections are prevented. This can be managed using oral hygiene gels that contain chlorohexidine, designed for dental care.

The procedure for the removal of the gastrostomy tube in animals over 10 kgs is to cut the catheter off flush with the skin after pulling it Taut. The catheter tip is

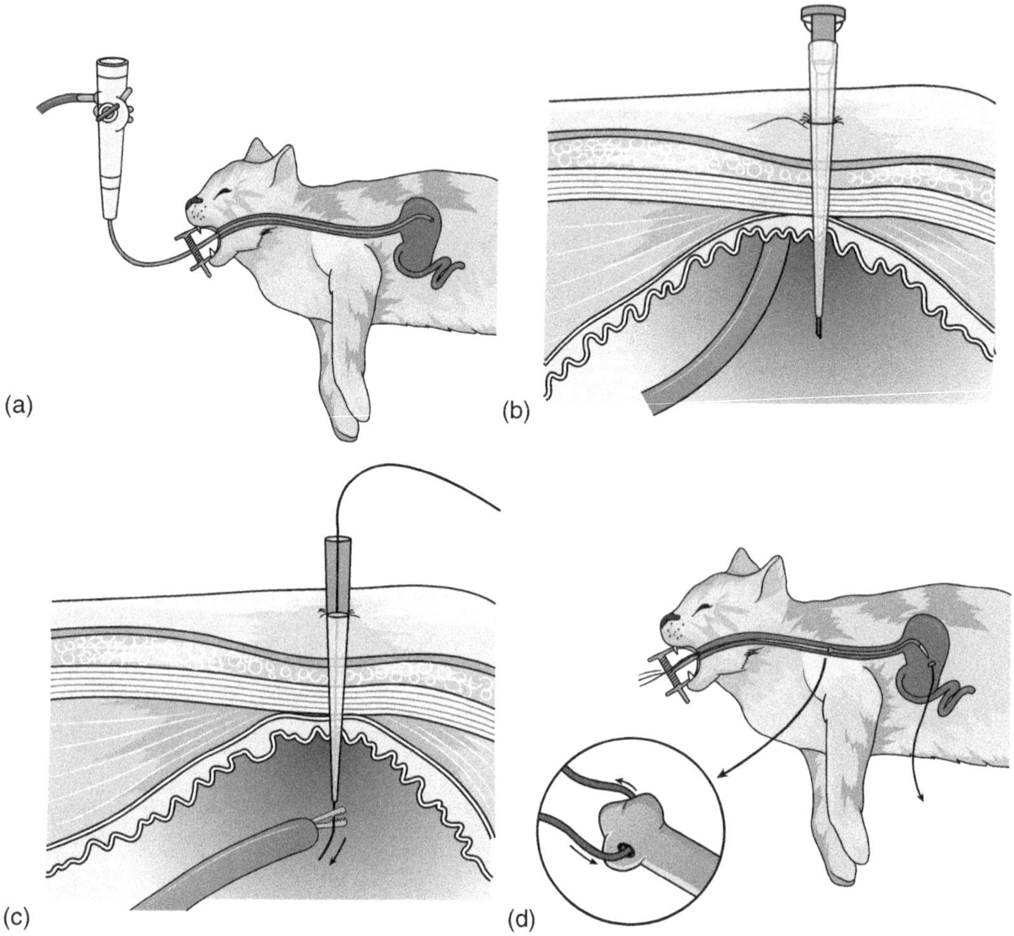

FIGURE 9.7 Placement of a PEG tube. (a) The animal should be placed in right lateral recumbency. The stomach is then insufflated with air introduced by the endoscope. The gastric wall will then become in contact with the body wall. (b) The lighted tip of the endoscope can be seen when pressed against the abdominal wall. This area should be prepared and scrubbed aseptically. A large-bore needle or over-the-needle catheter is inserted into the stomach next to the endoscope tip. (c) A thick nylon suture is fed through the needle or catheter, and is grasped by the endoscope's retrieval forceps. As the endoscope is withdrawn, the nylon suture is pulled out through the mouth. (d) The next stage is dependent on the type of tube used. To allow the feeding tube to be pulled through attached. Some commercial kits already have a catheter guide in place. The lubricated catheter (with attached feeding tube) is drawn down the oesophagus into the stomach by the suture which is exiting the body wall. (e) When the lubricated catheter guide reaches the body wall, resistance will be felt. Firm application of counter-pressure to the body wall should allow the catheter tip to emerge through the skin. In order for the feeding tube to exit, a very small incision (203mm) may be required. (f) As the feeding tube is pulled through, gentle traction will be required in order to bring the stomach and abdominal wall into close contact. A rubber/silicon flange slides down the tube and is secured in place.

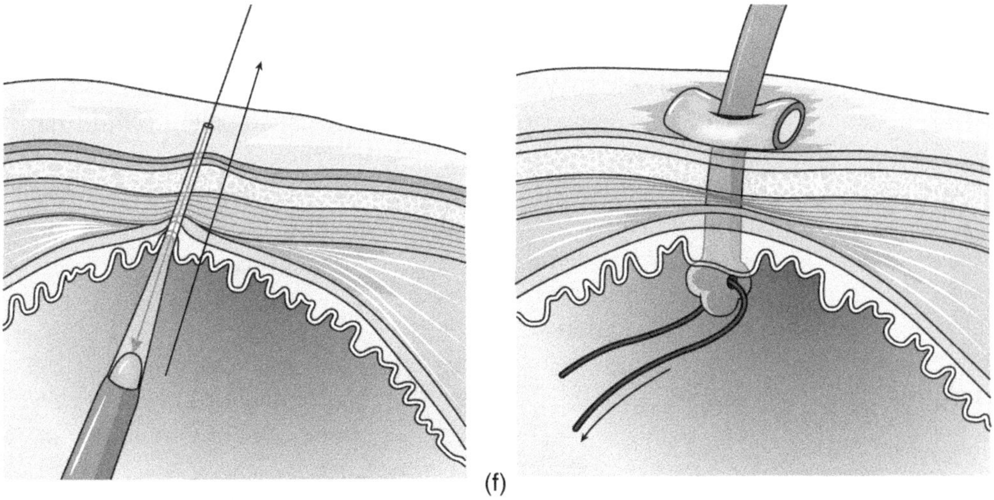

(e) (f)

FIGURE 9.7 (Continued)

then passed in the faeces. The resulting gastro-cutaneous fistula will rapidly heal if kept clean.

Delivery method	Common indications	Precautions
Nasogastric/ orogastric	• Unable to consume oral nutrition (e.g. intubated, sedated, neurologically impaired)	• Tube must be secured
	• Hypermetabolism in the presence of functional GIT (e.g. burns)	• Verify placement of tube by blue litmus method or by X-ray
Nasoduodenal/ nasojejunal	• Inadequate gastric motility (e.g. gastroparesis)	• Tube must be secured
	• Partial gastric outlet obstruction	• Verify placement of tube by X-ray or endoscopically
	• Severe aspiration risk	• Potential dumping syndrome
	• Oesophageal reflex	
	• After upper GI surgery	
Gastrotomy	• Anyone who requires medium to long-term NG tube feeding (> 1 month)	• Caution in patients with severe GE reflux or gastroparesis
• Percutaneous endoscopic (PEG)	• Head and neck injury/surgery	• Contraindicated in patients with ascites and coagulopathies
• Radiological		
• Surgical		
Jejunostomy	• Injury, obstruction or fistula proximal to the jejunum	• Potential dumping syndrome
• PEJ		
• Surgical		

(Continued)

	Advantages	Disadvantages
Enteral feeding	Nutrition getting to the enterocytes and colonocytes Nutrition is being supplied to the GI biome More physiological Simple/cheaper No central line required Less monitoring Less complications	Dependent on the gastrointestinal system working Adverse reactions (vomiting, diarrhoea) Food intolerance (psychological) Feeding tube complications Aspirations.
Parenteral feeding	Independent of gastrointestinal functioning	Nonphysiological Required central venous access Higher risk of systemic infection Cost More complications

KEY POINTS

Always perform a nutritional assessment on every patient, every time, to ensure adequate nutrition is being achieved.

RER calculations only calculate the number of calories to be fed; they don't take into consideration nutrients.

Always consider assisted tube feeding as an option.

FURTHER READING

Chan, D.L. (ed.) (2015). *Nutritional Management of Hospitalized Small Animals*. Chichester, UK: Wiley Blackwell.

REFERENCES

1. Freeman, L., Becvarova, I., Cave, N. et al. (2011). WSAVA nutritional assessment guidelines. *J. Small Anim. Pract.* 52 (7): 385–396.
2. Chan, D. (2005). Parenteral nutritional support. In: *Textbook of Veterinary Internal Medicine*, 6e, vol. 1 (ed. S.J. Ettinger and E.C. Feldman), 586–591. Missouri: Elsevier Science.
3. Remillard, R.L., Armstrong, P.J., and Davenport, D.J. (2000). Assisted feeding in hospitalised patients: enteral and parenteral nutrition. In: *Small Animal Clinical Nutrition*, 4e (ed. M.S. Hand, C.D. Thatcher, R.L. Remillard, and P. Roudebush), 351–399. Missouri: Mark Morris Institute.
4. Michel, K.E. (2006). Deciding who needs nutritional support. *Waltham Focus* 16 (3): 17–21.
5. Philpott, D.J., McKay, D.M., and Mak, W. (1998). Signal transduction pathways involved in enterohemorrhagic *Escherichia coli*-induced alterations in T84 epithelial permeability. *Infect. Immun.* 66: 1680–1687.

6. Cave, N.J. (2006). Hydrolysed protein diets for dogs and cats. *Vet. Clin. N. Am. Small Anim. Pract.* 36: 1251–1268.
7. Elliott, D.A. (2015). Nutritional support in acute kidney injury in dogs and cats. In: *Nutritional Management of Hospitalized Small Animals* (ed. D. Chan). Chichester, UK: Wiley Blackwell.
8. Becvarova, I. (2015). Tube feeding in small animals: diet selection and preparation. In: *Nutritional Management of Hospitalized Small Animals* (ed. D. Chan). Chichester, UK: Wiley Blackwell.
9. Gajanayake, I. (2015). Nasoesophageal feeding tubes in dogs and cats. In: *Nutritional Management of Hospitalized Small Animals* (ed. D. Chan). Chichester, UK: Wiley Blackwell.
10. Department of Diabetes, Endocrinology, Nutritional Medicine and Metabolism, Inselspital, Bern University Hospital, and University of Bern. http://www.udem.insel.ch/de/lehre-und-forschung/forschung/wichtige-abbildungen/ (accessed 26 February 2026).
11. Friedli, N., Stanga, Z., Culkin, A. et al. (2018). Management and prevention of refeeding syndrome in medical inpatients: an evidence-based and consensus-supported algorithm. *Nutrition* 2018 (47): 13–20.
12. Buffington, T., Holloway, C., and Abood, S. (2004). *Manual of Veterinary Dietetics*. Missouri: Elsevier Saunders.

CHAPTER 10

Cognitive Dysfunction

Cognitive dysfunction describes geriatric or senior behavioural changes, which are not solely attributed to a general medical condition, such as infection, organ failure or neoplasm [1]. Other terms, such as senile dementia and senile degeneration of the brain, are also often used. It should be remembered that cognitive dysfunction should not be considered a normal process of 'getting old'. It is rather a pathological condition that can result from encephalitis, tumours or other structural diseases, metabolic conditions (e.g. hypothyroidism) or idiopathic conditions. Owners may not present their dog or cat to the practice necessarily for behavioural or cognitive changes, but on questioning and clinical history taking, the clinical signs might become evident.

Aims of clinical nutrition for pets suffering from cognitive dysfunction include:

- Aid in reducing the behavioural changes associated with cognitive dysfunction.
- Feed a nutritionally balanced diet aimed at the senior life stage. Whilst maintaining an ideal body and muscle condition score.
- Aim to reduce the oxidative stress by neutralising free radicals and thus preventing extensive cellular damage.

CLINICAL NUTRITION

Proteins

The protein levels in diets aimed at animals with cognitive dysfunction need to be at similar levels as senior life-stage diets. Levels tend to be around 19–20% (DMB). This is to aid in maintaining heart and kidney health in the senior animal. Though there are no specified nutrient levels for senior pets, assumptions are made regarding protein levels. Protein should be of good quality (biological value) and not in excess.

Carbohydrates

The levels of carbohydrates within the diet do need to reflect that the senior animal can be less active than adults. The calorific levels of carbohydrate content can therefore be decreased. It is recommended, though, that the fibre content of senior diets be higher than that of adult life-stage diets. Bowel function in older dogs can be decreased, and the addition of fibre can assist in its functioning. Carbohydrate (NFE) levels are recommended at around 55% (DMB), and crude fibre at 4.5% (DMB). The role of fibres (prebiotics) is discussed in Chapter 6.

Fats

The overall level of fats within the diet does need to reflect a senior diet. The type of fats contained within the diet is important. Levels of the omega-3 fatty acids docosahexaenoic acid (DHA) and eicosapentaenoic acid (EPA) need to be increased. These fats contribute to neuronal cell membrane plasticity and health [2]. The decline in structural and functional integrity of the brain tissue correlates with the loss of DHA concentrations from the cell membranes. The brain is rich in polyunsaturated fatty acids (PUFAs), especially DHA, concentrations of PUFAs directly reflecting the concentrations within the diet. It has therefore been concluded that diets with increased levels of n-6 and n-3 fatty acids may help to delay or reduce the onset of neurodegenerative disorders such as cognitive dysfunction [2].

The main PUFAs of interest are DHA, EPA and arachidonic acid (ARA) [3]. Both ARA and DHA are the major constituents of the brain phospholipid membrane, can act as an immune suppressant and induce inflammatory responses, blood clotting, and cell signalling [4–6]. DHA has also been shown to protect against neurodegenerative diseases such as Alzheimer's and Parkinson's, as well as multiple sclerosis [7]. EPA and DHA (n-3) play an important role in the cardiovascular system and in treating psychiatric disorders [8]. There has been a very small amount of research looking at medium-chain triglycerides in dogs and their role in neuroprotective elements; as of yet, this hasn't been replicated in cats [9].

Vitamins and Minerals

The levels of the vitamins and minerals, which act as antioxidants, are increased in diets aimed at dogs with cognitive dysfunction. This is due to the effects that the antioxidants have on protecting against free radical damage. The main antioxidants used are vitamins E and C, beta-carotene and selenium. Vitamin E is used to help neutralise free radical reactivity. Antioxidants are believed to promote recovery in neurons that are exhibiting signs of neuropathology, and therefore, nutritional manipulation is believed to offer useful medication-related treatments for cognitive dysfunction. Vitamin C regenerates vitamin E, restoring its antioxidant activity. Beta-carotene reinforces vitamin E and also boosts its antioxidant capacity. Selenium in the diet aids by being a component of the antioxidant enzyme glutathione peroxidase.

The levels of other vitamins and minerals within the diet need to reflect the levels required by animals at a senior life stage.

FEEDING A DOG WITH COGNITIVE DYSFUNCTION

Diets have been designed to encompass all of these nutritional components. The difficulty arises when the animal is suffering from another disease or disorder that also requires a clinical diet specifically for this problem. Supplements have been designed that contain the antioxidants recommended for cognitive dysfunction. The levels of fatty acids in the diet can be achieved by using oil supplements; these supplements do need to be kept in an air-tight container to prevent oxidation of the fats.

As diets aimed at cognitive dysfunction are based on a senior life-stage diet, there are very few side effects experienced when changing to these diets. It should be remembered that older dogs can be fussier with their diets, and transitioning to a new diet can be difficult. It should also be noted to owners that there is no cure for cognitive dysfunction, only aid in delaying some of the symptoms. Regular examinations at the veterinary practice should be advocated, along with medications if required.

Mental stimulation in older dogs and cats is vital to maintaining cognitive function. The use of food to help in this stimulation can be key, with the use of puzzle feeders aiding in enrichment. New puzzles and enrichment methods should be introduced slowly and at a base level. Many animals' interactions will be slow to start and might need more encouragement from the owner than younger ones, but they should still be advocated.

REFERENCES

1. Frank D. (2000). Cognitive dysfunction in dogs. *Hill's European Symposium on Canine Brain Ageing*, 22–27.
2. Youdim, K.A., Martin, A., and Joseph, J.A. (2000). Essential fatty acids and the brain: possible health implications. *Int. J. Dev. Neurosci.* 18: 383–399.
3. Shanab, S.M.M., Hafez, R.M., and Fouad, A.S. (2018). A review on algae and plants as potential source of arachidonic acid. *J. Adv. Res.* 11: 3–13.
4. Hansen, J. and Schape, D. (1997). Docosahexaenoic acid plus arachidonic acid enhance preterm infant growth. *Prostaglandins Leukot. Essent. Fatty Acids* 57 (196).
5. Kinsella, J.E., Lokesh, B., Broughton, S., and Whelan, J. (2010). Dietary polyunsaturated fatty acids and eicosanoids: potential effects on the modulation of inflammatory and immune cells: an overview. *Nutrition* 6: 24–44.
6. Neitzel, J.J. (2010). Fatty acid molecules: fundamentals and role in signaling. *Nat. Educ.* 3 (9): 57.
7. Valenzuela, R., Sanhueza, J., and Valenzuela, A. (2012). Docosahexaenoic acid (DHA), and important fatty acid in aging and the protection of neurodegenerative diseases. *J. Nutr. Ther.* 1: 63–72.
8. Hallahan, B. and Garland, M.R. (2015). Essential fatty acids and mental health. *Br. J. Psychiatry* 186: 275–277.
9. Pan, Y., Larson, B., Araujo, J.A. et al. (2010). Dietary supplementation with medium-chained TAG has long-lasting cognition-enhancing effects in aged dogs. *Br. J. Nutr.* 103 (12): 1746–1754.

CHAPTER 11

Dental Nutrition

The incidence of dental disease shows that it is the most common problem adult dogs and cats suffer from. Incident rates of 85% of dogs and 70% of cats over the age of three suffer from some form of dental disease [1]. The development of periodontal disease depends on the host's immunity and inflammatory responses to plaque on the tooth's surface [2].

The aim of nutrition for dental issues includes:

- Encouraging chewing; this can be achieved by using kibbles of different sizes.
- Limiting the components of plaque and the mineralisation of plaque to tartar.
- Encourage the correct biome within the oral cavity to help prevent the formation of biofilms.

Plaque begins reforming rapidly within 4–12 hours after brushing, highlighting the need for daily, consistent oral hygiene. Bacteria in the mouth mix with saliva and food debris, settling on the enamel surface to form a biofilm. Bacteria feed on carbohydrates, producing acids that not only contribute to plaque formation but also cause tooth decay (mainly in humans). If this biofilm and plaque are not removed by brushing or other mechanical means, the plaque can harden into tartar (calculus) via mineralisation with calcium within 24 to 72 hours, which requires dental hygiene (descaling) treatment to remove.

CLINICAL NUTRITION

The diet of the animal can play an important preventive and therapeutic role. The type of food consumed, its texture and composition directly affect the oral environment. The use of these diets and their overall effectiveness depend on three factors.

1. The level of plaque present on the teeth and the animal's response to the plaque on the teeth (gingivitis).
2. The owner's ability to accomplish dental home care on the pet (e.g. tooth brushing).

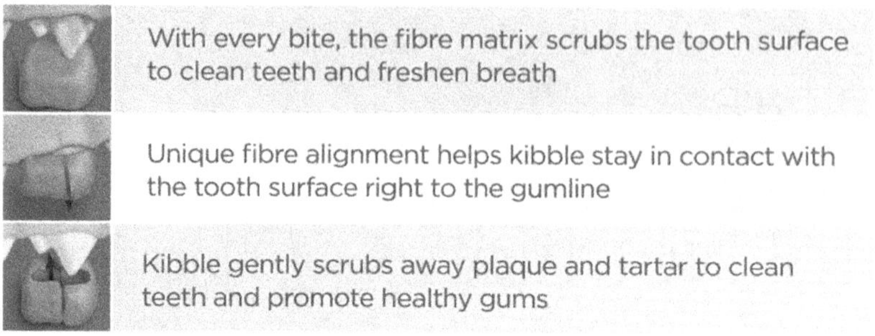

FIGURE 11.1 Soft kibbles with aligned fibres create a physical mechanism of 'wiping' off the plaque.

3. The selection of the methods of oral home care by the veterinary practice for the owner. Consideration should include products that are most likely to ensure compliance; this also includes the cost of the products.

Dental diets are designed with a few different mechanisms. The kibble size is influential; larger kibbles force the animal to chew the kibble, increasing chewing activity. The textures of the diet, as with those that are high in fibre, are beneficial in the removal of plaque and calculus from the teeth (Figure 11.1). Calculus is formed by the mineralisation of plaque by, in particular, calcium. Calcium is secreted in the saliva and is thus part of the reason why certain teeth have larger calcium deposits; these teeth tend to be located next to salivary ducts. The use of polyphosphates in the diet or supplements is to bind the calcium from the saliva, making it unavailable for the formation of calculus. The calcium is then released as normal in the digestive tract and absorbed by the animal. The use of polyphosphates is more effective when coating the kibble rather than being incorporated into the kibble [2].

Carbohydrates

The use of fibres specifically aligned within the kibble is proven to reduce plaque and calculus formation accumulating on the tooth. But other forms of carbohydrates in high levels can be detrimental. The oral biome bacteria utilise fermentable carbohydrates, like glucose, as a source of energy and create biofilms and plaque more readily. Caries can form as a by-product of this process. This is because the by-products of carbohydrate fermentation are acidic and cause demineralisation of the enamel [3]. Changes in the diet, along with dental home care, can prevent the formation of caries in dogs. Caries in the cat are exceptionally rare but have been reported [3].

Protein

A diet deficient in protein has been shown to cause degenerative changes in the periodontium. Periodontium is defined as the tissues surrounding the tooth, which include the gingiva, the periodontal ligament and the alveolus; in some contexts, the cement is

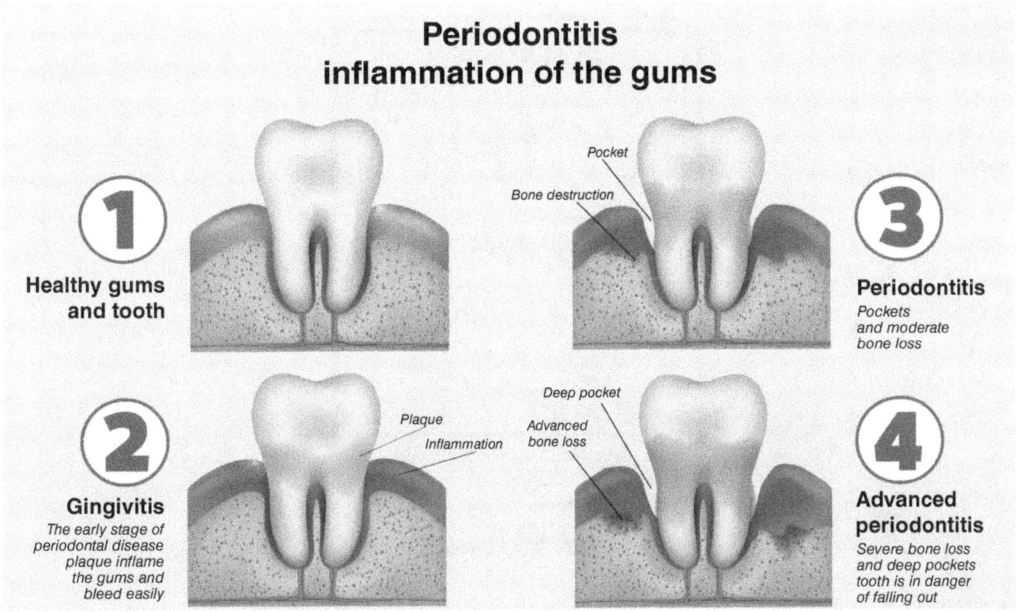

FIGURE 11.2 Demonstration of the progression of periodontal disease.

also considered part of the periodontium. As protein deficiencies rarely occur in dogs and cats as a typical cause of periodontal disease, it is not a practical consideration. In some diets, protein levels are moderately reduced to limit the components of plaque (Figure 11.2).

Vitamins and Minerals

Calcium and phosphorus consumed in unbalanced ratios can lead to secondary nutritional hyperparathyroidism and significant loss of alveolar bone. The loss of bone can support the progression of periodontitis. Moderately reducing the levels of calcium in the diet, or its availability, can help limit the mineralisation of plaque to tartar. The addition of polyphosphates (calcium chelating agents) can produce a significant reduction in tartar formation (~45%) [4]. Zinc has both antibacterial and healing properties (promotes a healthy epithelium) [5]. Zinc salts can also inhibit the formation of tartar (calculus).

Vitamins C and A can also aid in dental problems and are sometimes supplemented in dental diets. Vitamin C is important in the production of collagen, which is the main protein found within the gums. Vitamin A aids in protecting the epithelium.

FEEDING A DENTAL DIET

The use of diets is aimed primarily at preventing and removing small amounts of plaque and calculus. If the animal has larger amounts of calculus or periodontal disease, dental descaling and polishing will be required. Prophylactic diets, chews and

FIGURE 11.3 Example of the Veterinary Oral Health Council logo.

tooth brushing can be recommended post-dentistry. Most diets designed for dentistry are based around a senior life-stage diet, and those animals which require a diet with a high energy density may require additional calories from another source. Dental diets are poor at removing plaque from the subgingival area, and dental hygiene procedures (subgingival planning) will still be required to remove this debris.

The uses of dental hygiene chews are widely used, mainly due to the ease of compliance. Owners love the idea that they are giving their pet a treat, alongside it being a preventive treatment. Guidance does need to be followed with the use of these dental chews. Chews that are based on a rice flour formula and have a calorific value. Manufacturer's guidelines state that a portion of the daily food ration needs to be removed if a chew is given.

Finding dental diets and chews that are clinically effective can be difficult, as many products state that they aid in dental health but may have limited clinical evidence supporting this claim. The Veterinary Oral Health Council (VOHC) ensures that there is peer-reviewed evidence for the specific product and will permit its logo to be displayed on the packaging. These studies are reviewed by a board of veterinary dental specialists. Approval is only granted if the evidence is of a specific standard (Figure 11.3).

DENTAL SUPPLEMENTS

There are many supplement products that are available on the market that aid in dental health. Look for the VOHC logo to ensure that there is clinical evidence behind the product. Some utilise a specific seaweed (*Ascophyllum nodosum*) that works systemically by being ingested and absorbed into the bloodstream, which alters the saliva composition to soften existing plaque and tartar. It prevents new, hard tartar from adhering to teeth, reducing bad breath and improving overall dental hygiene within three to eight weeks of daily use.

REFERENCES

1. Stiefel, D.J., Truelove, E.L., Chin, M.M., and Mandel, L.S. (1992). Efficacy of chlorhexidine swabbing in oral health care for people with severe disabilities. *Spec Care Dentist* 12 (2): 57–62.
2. Furniss, G. (2006). The role of nutrition in the dental care of dogs and cats. *Vet. Rev.* 114: 50–54.
3. Tutt, C. (2006). Tooth friendly diets. *UK Vet.* 11 (6): 78–80.
4. Gorrel, C. and Derbyshire, S. (2005). *Veterinary Dentistry for the Nurse and Technician.* Oxford: Elsevier Butterworth Heinemann.
5. Servet, E., Hendriks, W., and Clarke, D. (2003). Taking care of cats' teeth – kibbles can be useful in the prevention of periodontal disease. *Waltham Focus* 13 (3): 32–35.

CHAPTER 12

Dermatological Disease

The terms food allergy and food hypersensitivity should be reserved for those adverse reactions to food that have an immunologic basis. Food intolerance refers to adverse food reactions (AFRs) due to non-immunologic mechanisms. Dermatologists suggest that only 1–6% of all dermatoses seen in practice relate to AFRs and that food allergies constitute 10–20% of allergic responses in dogs and cats [1] (Figure 12.1). A full dermatological workup is required before a nutritional factor can be entirely confirmed. It can be commonplace, however, for owners to self-diagnose their pet's food allergy or intolerance, even before seeing the veterinary surgeon. There are many diets available that are gluten-free, grain-free, hypoallergenic and/or natural, and when the pet improves on these diets, the owners assume that their pet has an allergy or intolerance to one of the ingredients.

The skin is the largest organ of the body and has a heavy demand on bodily nutrient supply. When factors become suboptimal, it is usually the skin that becomes the first organ to demonstrate deterioration. The owner can easily detect signs of deterioration, loss of coat sheen and coat shedding, and the coat can become greasy, and scurf at the skin surface can be evident, but in many cases, the signs of deterioration occur at such a slow rate that owners don't notice (Table 12.1). It is not until the issue is resolved, or the animal is placed on a different diet, that the animal's coat returns to 'healthy' and the owner notices a difference.

The correct levels of fats and proteins within the diet are important to maintain the integrity of the cell membranes, which are comprised of a phospholipid bilayer (Figure 12.2).

Food intolerance is not so clear-cut and is a more controversial area. Although not life-threatening, it can and often does make the sufferer feel extremely unwell and can have a major impact on life. Some people (and other mammals) lack the enzymes needed to break foods down, for example, lactose intolerance, where the enzyme lactase is not produced in large enough amounts to break down the lactose (milk sugars) in milk. Food intolerance reactions do not involve immunoglobulin E (IgE), and the mechanisms are unclear; however, it is known that reactions are more likely to be delayed, with the reaction occurring several hours and sometimes

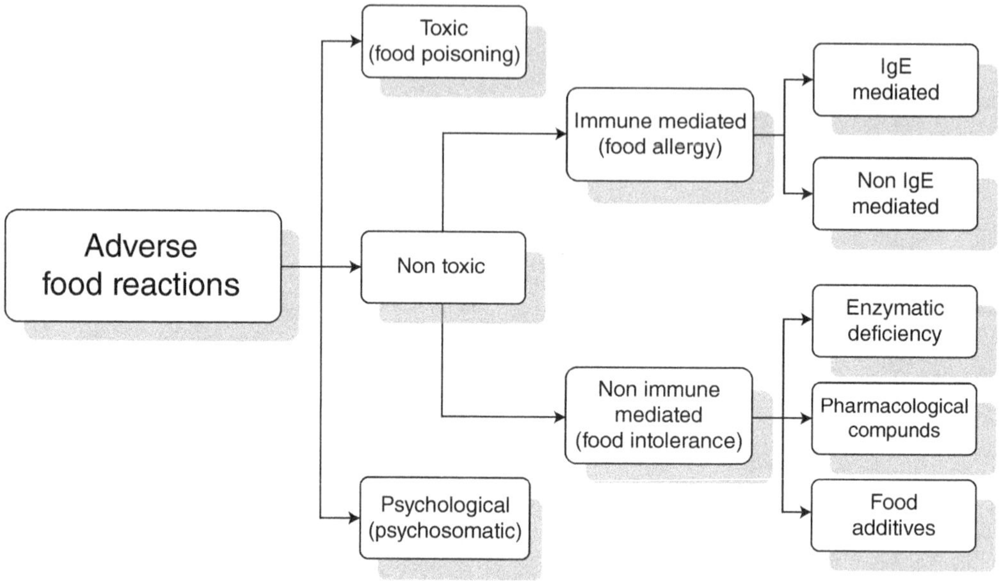

FIGURE 12.1 Adverse food reactions (AFRs) classifications.

TABLE 12.1 Deficiencies and their effect on the skin in the dog.

Nutrient elements	Function concerning the skin and coat	Minimum canine requirement (per MJ)	Clinical signs of insufficiency
Protein	Structure and pigment of keratinocytes and hair, components of sebum and sweat	9.6 g	Depigmentation of skin and hair, dry coat and hair loss
Lipids	Energy, precursors of eicosanoids, components of membrane phospholipids	3.3 g	Dull, dry coat, alopecia, greasy skin and pruritus
Linoleic acid	Maintenance of an effective cutaneous barrier	0.66 g	Dry, scaly skin
Zinc	Metalloenzyme component, RNA and DNA polymerase cofactor	3.0 mg	Crusting/scaling of skin, erythema and alopecia
Copper	Melanin and keratinocyte synthesis	0.3 mg	Hypopigmentation and a dry, rough coat
Vitamin E	Antioxidant, stabiliser of cell membranes	1.8 IU	Scale, erythema and alopecia
Vitamin A	Cell growth and differentiation, the keratinisation process	245.5 IU	Hyperkeratinisation, scaling and alopecia
Biotin	Metabolic enzyme cofactor	—	Facial alopecia and crusting
Riboflavin	Metabolic enzyme cofactor	0.15 mg	Dry, flaky dermatitis, swollen and cracked lips
Niacin	Metabolic enzyme cofactor	0.72 mg	Pruritic dermatitis
Pyridoxine	Metabolic enzyme cofactor	0.07 mg	Dull, waxy coat and facial alopecia

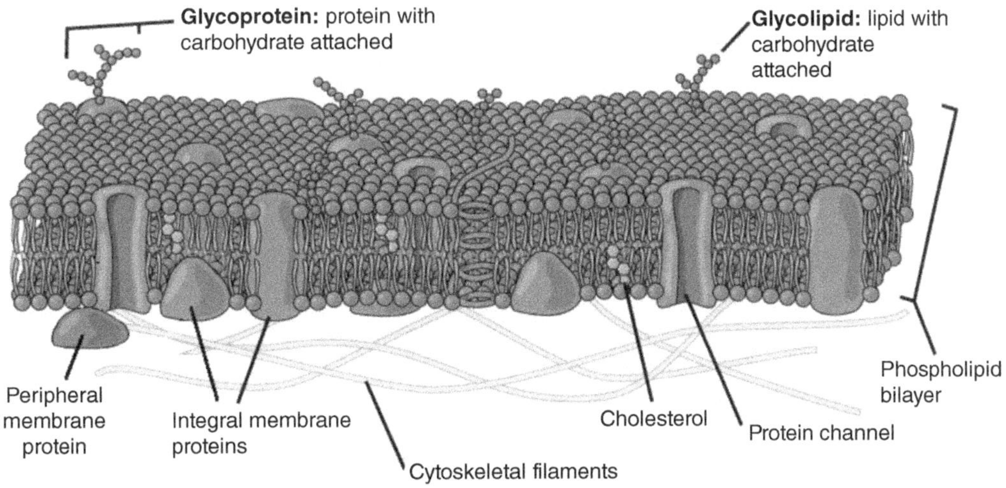

FIGURE 12.2 Diagrammatic representation of cell membranes.

up to several days after eating the offending food. The symptoms caused by these reactions are numerous but have been associated with gut symptoms such as bloating, diarrhoea, constipation and IBS, and skin problems such as eczema [2]. Specific food additives, which are known to cause problems, include onions and propylene glycol, which can cause haematological abnormalities in cats. Lactose intolerance is a relatively common metabolic adverse reaction in dogs and cats [3]. Diarrhoea can develop when given cows' or even goats' milk, due to the lactose content being higher than that of bitch's or queen's milk [4]. Gluten-sensitive enteropathy has been well documented in Irish Setters [5].

Aims of nutritional management include:

- Help to avoid common food allergens.
- Using a highly digestible diet helps limit the amount of undigested protein passing through to the gastrointestinal tract, which could provoke an allergic reaction.
- Discuss with clients how to conduct an effective food trial and the necessity to comply with strict restrictions. This also includes food hygiene requirements.

CLINICAL NUTRITION

Fats

A common recommendation for atopic dermatitis is the supplementation of the diet with omega (n)−3 essential fatty acids (EFAs). Dietary supplementation has been shown to normalise the cutaneous fatty acid profile and improve the clinical signs in dogs with seborrhoea. EFAs fulfil several roles in the body and skin. These include binding water into the stratum corneum, forming the epidermal permeability barrier, acting as antioxidants and providing substrate for eicosanoids such as prostaglandin and leukotrienes. n−3 fatty acids compete with those of the n−6 series for the same

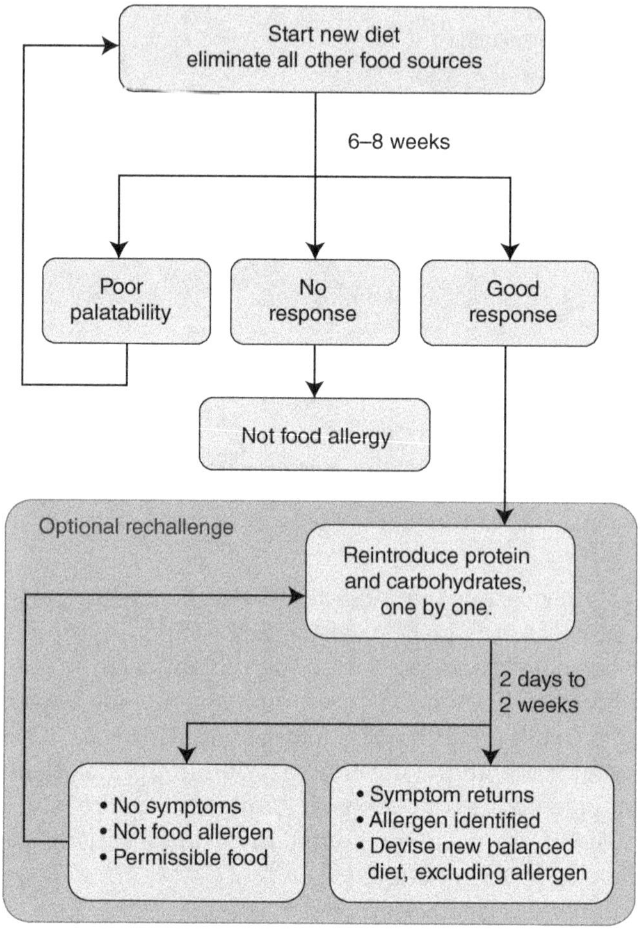

FIGURE 12.3 Protocol for food elimination trial.

enzymes, so n−3 supplementation will inhibit the formation of arachidonic acid and its proinflammatory metabolites [3] (Figure 12.3). Traditionally, dermatological diets and supplements were quoted as needing fatty acids in the correct ratio of n−6:n−3 fatty acids to be between 5:1 and 10:1 for the dog [4]. Fatty acid supplements that are commonly administered include starflower/borage, evening primrose and corn oils, which are high in levels of omega-6 EFAs. Cold-water marine fish, algae, meat, linseed and soya contain levels of omega-3 EFAs. In many diets and supplements now, omega-6 EFAs are no longer being supplemented. Omega-6 EFAs are primarily required in the role of repair for cell membranes, and the amount found in the diet will be sufficient for this role, without the requirement for supplementation. The omega-6 EFAs have been shown to harm the reduction of inflammation.

Palmitoylethanolamide (PEA) is a naturally occurring bioactive lipid and endocannabinoid-like molecule produced on demand by damaged exposed cells. PEA has been shown to counteract inflammation, itch, and pain (including neuropathic) [6]. PEA's role in canine and feline dermatitis is just starting to be investigated, but it is showing some positive effects.

Vitamins and Minerals

Vitamin deficiencies are rarely diagnosed, and due to the large quantity of animals being fed a commercially balanced diet, it is unlikely. Any deficiencies are more likely to be a consequence of a genetic enzyme defect or an absorption problem. Vitamin deficiencies may occur in animals receiving a fat-restricted diet or having poor fat absorption. Some dietary components can also inactivate specific vitamins. For example, avidin in raw egg whites will bind biotin. Excessive amounts of the water-soluble vitamins can also be lost if the animal is suffering from polyuria. Vitamin A-responsive dermatosis is entirely confined to Cocker Spaniels and is a rare condition. The condition is characterised by focal areas of follicular plugging with accumulation of keratin. Daily doses of 10,000 IU of vitamin A are required to resolve these lesions [5].

Zinc deficiencies, when an absolute dietary deficiency is present, are considered rare. More commonly, there is a relative deficiency due to interaction or an inability to utilise the ingested zinc. Absorption can be inhibited by iron, copper and calcium and reduced by intestinal phytate and inorganic phosphate. Calcium, iron and copper all compete with zinc absorption. Animals that receive high levels of calcium in their diet are more likely to present with zinc deficiencies. These animals tend to be large or giant breeds, which receive over-supplementation of calcium during growth periods. Specific breeds, such as Siberian Huskies and Alaskan Malamutes, appear to be unable to absorb adequate quantities of zinc. Bull Terriers can suffer from lethal acrodermatitis, a metabolic inability to utilise zinc. This can result in systemic signs such as emaciation, stunting and immunocompetence. Zinc supplementation with oral zinc sulphate at 10 mg/kg bwt, or zinc methionate at 1.7 mg/kg bwt once daily with food, is the treatment of choice for the breed [5]. Supplementation for other breeds may be required for the period until any dermatological lesions resolve, provided that the animal is placed on a nutritionally balanced complete diet. Some may require lifelong supplementation.

Proteins

When designing or recommending an elimination diet, certain characteristics need to be taken into consideration. A limited number of protein sources are required, along with the protein being from a novel source. Excessive levels of protein should be avoided; the protein present needs to be of a digestibility greater than 87%. The use of hydrolysed protein can be used, as its digestibility is high. Digestibility is an important factor, as free amino acids and small peptides make poor antigens. The diet needs to be free of additives and excessive levels of vasoactive amines whilst still being nutritionally adequate for the animal's life stage and body score.

Hydrolysed diets are advantageous as they remove the absolute necessity of finding the primary causal agent of the food allergen. Hydrolysed diets work by taking a protein and reducing it in size through hydrolysis. When the hydrolysed protein is then ingested, the body no longer recognises the protein as an antigen, and the allergic immune response is not initiated.

Carbohydrates

The use of carbohydrates in the diet also needs to be limited. In many elimination diets, the use of a novel carbohydrate source is also used. Many carbohydrate sources used include rice, sweet potato, white potato, and tapioca.

Elimination Food Trails

The use of elimination trials is an important aspect of the diagnosis and treatment/management of AFRs. Due to the length of time required for these food trials, owners must be fully educated in the criteria of the trial – an excellent role for the veterinary nurse/technician. Finding a novel diet for utilisation in the trial can be difficult and provides an excellent role for hydrolysed diets. Owners need to be aware of the most common mistakes that occur during the food trial; these include not feeding any other foods, including those of the same protein source; storage of the diet; cleaning of utensils; the length of the trial and restarting time frames if the pet does consume something it shouldn't (Figure 12.3).

Dietary-induced skin problems include food intolerances, primary and secondary nutrient deficiencies and nutrient toxicities. These are commonly grouped and termed AFRs. A full dietary history needs to be obtained, and owners should include all commercial foods, all snacks and treats, supplements, chewable/palatable medications and vitamins, chew toys, human foods and any food that the animal may have access to at any point in their life. Actively encourage owners to keep a food diary, as with obese animals and diabetics. The classification and diagnosis of nutrition-related skin disorders are initially based on a detailed dietary history and food evaluation. Veterinary nurses and technicians are in an ideal position to help owners make an accurate representation of what the pet consumes, educate owners, and help in compliance and concordance in the elimination food trial period.

INSECT PROTEIN

Insect protein is a highly digestible, sustainable and hypoallergenic alternative for dogs with dermatitis or food allergies, often reducing itching and skin irritations. Studies show significant improvement in skin health and gastrointestinal symptoms, making it a viable option for elimination diets. Common sources include black soldier fly larvae.

Elimination Diets

When designing or recommending an elimination diet, certain characteristics do need to be taken into consideration. Review the diet history sheets and diaries to give you an indication of what the animal has been exposed to in the past. A limited number of protein sources are required, along with the protein being from a novel source. Excessive levels of protein should be avoided; the protein present needs to be of a digestibility greater than 87%. The use of hydrolysed protein can be used, as its digestibility is high. Digestibility is an important factor as free amino acids and small peptides make poor antigens [6]. The diet needs to be free of additives and excessive levels of vasoactive amines whilst still being nutritionally adequate for the animal's life stage and body score.

Hydrolysed diets are advantageous as they remove the absolute necessity of finding the primary causal agent of the food allergen. Hydrolysed diets work by taking a protein and reducing it in size through hydrolysis. When the hydrolysed protein is then ingested, the body no longer recognises the protein as an antigen, and the allergic immune response is not initiated. The use of carbohydrates in the diet also needs to be limited. In many elimination diets, the use of a novel carbohydrate source is also utilised. Many carbohydrate sources used include rice, potato and tapioca.

Feeding an Elimination Food (Dermatological and Gastrointestinal Disease)

The main diagnosis method for nutritional AFRs is dietary elimination trials. Either a commercial product or a homemade diet can achieve these trials. It must be noted that homemade diets are likely to be nutritionally inadequate for maintenance requirements. Most homemade diets lack a source of calcium, EFAs, vitamins and other micronutrients. These diets can also contain excessive levels of protein. If the owner is insistent on the use of a homemade diet, guidance on constructing a balanced diet is required from the veterinary practice.

Common Mistake 1: Trying to Find Novel

To make a diagnosis of nutritional AFRs, only the elimination of food can be used. The trial needs to be performed for several weeks to months (12 weeks), and full dedication from the owner is required. The diet used as elimination diet requires to be a novel protein and carbohydrate source; a common mistake is that an inadequate diet history has been taken, the owner inadvertently forgetting previous exposure to certain ingredients or not even being aware of the ingredients within diets and treats fed previously, and thus, a protein or carbohydrate is used that isn't novel. Ensuring that the protein and carbohydrate source is novel can be very difficult. Lots of ingredients that owners might not recognise as having a protein source can also compromise elimination diets. For example, vegetables are not often viewed as a protein source, but have an excellent protein level. Use of a hydrolysed diet removes the requirement to find a diet that has a sole protein and carbohydrate source that is novel.

Common Mistake 2: Adding in Foods with the Same Novels

Elimination trials can prove to be extremely useful when diagnosing the causal nutritional agent in both dermatological and gastrointestinal diseases. A strict elimination trial protocol does need to be adhered to, and the owner and anyone in contact with the animal need to be aware of this. No other foodstuffs, other than the elimination food, should be ingested over this period. This includes treats, flavoured vitamins, chewable/palatable medications, fatty acid supplements and chew toys. Even if the additional foodstuffs are of the same novel protein or carbohydrate source or a hydrolysed protein, there can be differences in food additives, potential contaminations or additional other ingredients. Palatable tablets need to be changed to those without flavourings.

Common Mistake 3: Not Performing the Trial for Long Enough

Potential lengths of elimination trials must be clearly conveyed to the owner when initially discussing the trial; setting expectations of the length of the trial at the outset is important for compliance. The patient is fed the controlled elimination diet for up to 12 weeks for dermatological disease. A shorter period of two to four weeks can be satisfactory in gastrointestinal disease. The degree of clinical improvement during the elimination trial will be 100% only if food sensitivity is the sole causal agent. These trials are often difficult to interpret in dermatological disease. This is due to concurrent allergic skin disease. These patients may only partially respond to an elimination trial. Confirmation of a diagnosis can be made of an adverse food reaction when the clinical signs reoccur within 10–14 days after the animal is challenged with its original diet. Owners should be made aware that animals can have an AFR and an allergy to an environmental factor concurrently.

Common Mistake 4: Prolonged Elimination Can Build Tolerance

Weeks or months of elimination of the reactive food may well lead to reintroduction of the food without reaction. This is known as tolerance, and its maintenance depends on establishing the threshold of both frequency and quantity for that person – in other words, eating the food occasionally may be tolerated, but reintroducing it in large quantities or on a very regular basis (e.g. every day) might lead to symptoms recurring. Some misconceptions surround with the owner thinking the animal being misdiagnosed as having an AFR as when that food was reintroduced after a prolonged elimination, no adverse reaction is noted. No misdiagnosis had occurred, and tolerance was created.

Common Mistake 5: Storage/Dust Mite Contamination

Allergies to house dust and storage mites play an important role and are more significant than the pollens. Positive reactions to *Acarus* are seen in between 45 and 95% of atopic dogs, to *Typrophagus* in 60 and 89% and to *Dermatophagoides farinae* in 70 and 90%, depending on the literature source [7, 8]. 94% of dogs with atopic dermatitis had serum IgE against proteins from one or more of the storage mite species [7]. Many owners anecdotally report improvements in their dog's dermatological issues when changed from a dry commercial kibble to raw, frozen or wet diets. It has been demonstrated in 90% of studied dermatological diets that after five weeks of opening and storage, mites were evident [8]. The diets themselves, ingredients and nutrient composition were not the cause of the improvement, but rather the method of storage. Storage of the elimination diet is exceptionally important, alongside cleaning of food bowls and utensils involved in food preparation.

From an investigation into how to store dry commercial foods, recommendations are to keep dry diets in the original packaging and to use no more than a month's supply at a time [9]. The longer the food is broached, the higher the likelihood of mite contamination. Wet foods remove the potential for mite contamination, as do frozen foods.

AFRs cause a variety of clinical signs, from skin issues to gastrointestinal signs. A good diagnostic workup by the veterinary surgeon is required; part of this can include a food elimination trial. These trials can prove to be useful – but the interpretation of them can be difficult. Exceptionally good client guidance is needed in diet trials, and veterinary nurses/technicians should take a pivotal role in aiding clients.

Always give the client written instructions describing the requirements of the elimination trial and feeding quantities. Details on how to contact an advising veterinary nurse can prove useful if the owners have any questions during the trial.

REFERENCES

1. Gaschen, F.P. and Merchant, S.R. (2011). Adverse food reactions in dogs and cats. *Vet. Clin. North Am. Small Anim. Pract.* 41 (2): 361–379.
2. Craig, J.M. (2019). Food intolerance in dogs and cats. *J. Small Anim. Pract. 60* (2): 77–85.
3. Verlinden, A., Hesta, M., Millet, S., and Janssens, G.P.J. (2006). Food allergy in dogs and cats: a review. *Crit. Rev. Food Sci. Nutr.* 46 (3): 259–273.
4. Turnbull, J.L., Adams, H.N., and Gorard, D.A. (2014). Review article: the diagnosis and management of food allergy and food intolerances. *Aliment. Pharmacol. Ther.* 41 (1): 3–25.
5. Hall, E.J. and Batt, R.M. (1991). Abnormal permeability precedes the development of a gluten sensitive enteropathy in Irish setter dogs. *Gut* 32: 749–753.
6. Untersmayr, E. and Jensen-Jarolim, E. (2008). The role of protein digestibility and antacids on food allergy outcomes. *J. Allergy Clin. Immunol.* 121 (6): 1301–1308.
7. Arlian, L.G., Schumann, R.J., Morgan, M.S., and Glass, R.L. (2003). Serum immunoglobulin E against storage mite allergens in dogs with atopic dermatitis. *Am. J. Vet. Res.* 64 (1): 32–36.
8. Brazis, P., Serra, M., Sellés, A. et al. (2008). Evaluation of storage mite contamination of commercial dry dog food. *Vet. Dermatol.* 19: 209–214.
9. Gill, C., McEwan, N., McGarry, J., and Nuttall, T. (2011). House dust and storage mite contamination of dry dog food stored in open bags and sealed boxes in 10 domestic households. *Vet. Dermatol.* 22 (2): 162–172.

CHAPTER 13

Endocrine Disease

DIABETES MELLITUS

Introduction

Diabetes mellitus (DM) is a complex disease, with stabilisation of blood glucose levels being affected by confounding disease processes, efficacy of the primary disease control treatment, diet and exercise programmes and weight control. Thus, a full history of the animal, including all these factors, must be taken. There are several possible causes of DM, including pancreatitis, obesity, drugs (glucocorticoids and progestins), concurrent illness (hyperadrenocorticism (HAC) and acromegaly), genetics, immune-mediated insulitis, infections and islet amyloidosis. Obtaining an ideal body condition score in both cats and dogs is the ideal goal in all these cases, with obesity increasing the risk of DM in cats by fourfold. Obese diabetic animals may have difficulty losing weight, but the reduction of blood glucose levels is the initial aim, followed by a conservative weight loss programme, which does need to be carefully monitored by a veterinary professional.

Underweight animals, once stabilised, should be fed a modest increase in calories to promote repletion. Dietary therapy can help to improve glycaemic control, but emphasis should be placed on adjustment of the medication dosage and/or schedule and control of any other concurrent disease if present [1].

DIABETES TREATMENTS

With insulin-dependent DM, the beta cells within the pancreas lose their ability to secrete insulin, completely or partial reduction. This can be congenital or due to pancreatitis or prolonged disease of the pancreas [2]. The monitoring of pancreatic-specific enzymes should also occur when conducting routine monitoring of these cases, as it can be a primary cause. In cases when insulin resistance occurs at the site of the peripheral tissues, this can be referred to as Type 2 DM. The quantity of insulin secreted by the beta cells can be increased, decreased, or remain normal. In some texts, Type 2 diabetes, which resolves, is sometimes classed as transient Type 2 DM. This is more commonly noted in obese cats when insulin resistance becomes established. Once the cat obtains and then maintains an ideal body condition score, the hyperglycaemia can resolve, but the animal will still always have the potential to become hyperglycaemic again. If the beta cells also become exhausted, a period of exogenous insulin administration may be required. Hyperglycaemia is toxic to beta cells and aggravates the situation by further reducing insulin secretion. This mechanism can also explain why the more obese the animal and the longer that this animal has been obese, the greater the incidence of the onset of diabetes. Many factors can predispose the animal to insulin resistance.

Sodium-glucose cotransporter 2 (SGLT2) inhibitors are a newer class of orally administered medications for cats that inhibit glucose absorption from the kidney. Glucose is excreted in the urine, having the desired effect of lowering blood glucose levels.

CLINICAL NUTRITION

The nutritional aims that need to be considered when altering the diet of the animal include:

- Aid in the reduction of postprandial hyperglycaemic spikes.
- Maintain optimal body condition scores and hydration levels.
- Supply the required amounts of nutrients and calories for the specific life stage, including those lost through clinical symptoms (e.g. the water-soluble vitamins if polyuria (PU) is present).

Water

A clinical symptom of DM is polydipsia (PD) and PU. Obligatory losses of electrolytes, such as sodium, potassium, chloride, calcium and phosphorus and the water-soluble vitamins will occur. Access to fresh water at all times is required, and in severe cases, administration of parenteral fluid may be required. Monitoring fluid intake, if possible, is a good indicator of glucose control, and consequently medication effect if being administered. Diabetic diaries are a good idea, and if owners can comment on daily water consumption, this can be helpful when stabilising patients.

Proteins

The protein and carbohydrate ratio is an important factor in the clinical nutrition of diabetic cats. Protein levels in diabetic cats may need to be increased, especially in the quality of the provided proteins. This is due to losses of amino acids in the urine, a consequence of renal glomerulopathy or changes in hormonal signals. Excess protein levels need to be avoided, as renal damage can be enhanced.

In animals experiencing a loss of lean muscle mass due to the catabolism of protein for energy, muscle mass can be restored and increased following appropriate nutritional replenishment. The quantity and quality of the protein within the diet need to reflect this.

Carbohydrates

Consumption of soluble or simple carbohydrates is the primary cause of rapid postprandial hyperglycaemic spikes. Diets need to avoid high levels of soluble carbohydrates, and the feeding of treats high in soluble carbohydrates should be stopped. Use of insoluble carbohydrates, fibre, has a positive effect on glycaemic control in both dogs and cats. Diets that contain fibre, which exerts gelling properties, can slow the rate of presentation of nutrients (including glucose) to the body. This helps reduce the postprandial spike. The fermentation products of fibre, short-chain or volatile fatty acids, also modify the secretion of some of the digestive hormones and the sensitivity of tissues to insulin. Complex carbohydrates should provide ~50–60% of the calories in diets for dogs and in situations where cats are being fed a high-fibre diet [1].

Felines are obligate carnivores and have a unique metabolism. Initially, feeding a growth diet was the diet of choice due to the relative protein increase and decrease in carbohydrate content. Specific diets aimed at diabetic cats are widely available. In cases where owners are unable to afford a veterinary therapeutic diet, a good-quality kitten diet can still be recommended. A decrease in carbohydrate content will also create an increase in DM% of fat content. A high-protein and low-carbohydrate diet has been shown to enhance insulin sensitivity. This combination of high protein, low carbohydrate closely resembles the natural diet of a cat in the wild. Studies examining this dietary therapy have shown that insulin treatments could be discontinued in 15 out of 24 cats [3].

In cats receiving SGLT2 inhibitors, the initial research work on the pharmaceutical was conducted whilst the cats were fed a decreased carbohydrate diet [4]. Recommendations from the manufacturers are currently to perform a nutritional assessment on the patient and to feed accordingly.

Vitamins and Minerals

PU (a common clinical symptom of diabetes) will increase the loss of electrolytes and water-soluble vitamins, with magnesium and phosphorous being the most significantly lost. Chromium can be used to improve peripheral insulin sensitivity and glucose tolerance, though accurate studies on the use of chromium have not been conclusive.

Feeding a Diabetic Cat

On diagnosis of DM, a full nutritional assessment of the patient is required. A high carbohydrate diet should be avoided, as should semimoist diets. These diets have a hyperglycaemic effect due to the increased levels of simple carbohydrates and other ingredients used as humectants (e.g. glycerine). Cost does play a deciding factor in choosing a diet for a diabetic patient, as does whether the animal eats the food. An underweight animal will need a modified diet to gain weight, but this can only be achieved with management of the diabetes.

Administration of exogenous insulin does not necessarily need to be coordinated with times of feeding in cats. The owner needs to be aware of the detrimental effects of feeding snacks and treats that the veterinary surgeon responsible for the case is not aware of. Milk should also be avoided due to the calorific intake. The timing of meals is not as critical in feline diabetic patients, and it is advised to continue feeding the cat in the way that it is used to (e.g. free-choice feeding). Free-choice feeding is not the same as ad libitum feeding, where the animal has access to unlimited food. In free-choice feeding, only a set total daily amount is permitted, but as the name suggests, the animal has free choice when it chooses to eat the food. Twice-a-day feeding is not advocated in cats, unlike in dogs.

Cats that are being treated with SGLT2 inhibitors are recommended to be fed a diet that best reflects their body condition score. Whatever diet helps to obtain an ideal body condition score is advocated. At the time of writing, there has been no research based on the formulation of the diet being received in conjunction with this treatment regimen.

Several studies have investigated diet formulation (wet vs dry) and carbohydrate content of the diet. One study found that the remission rate was 29%, with a threefold higher chance of achieving remission for cats fed a commercial wet diet (low carbohydrate) compared to cats fed a diet with a moderate to high carbohydrate level. Remission is thought to occur as a result of the reversal of glucotoxicity [5, 6]. By lowering and stabilising postprandial blood glucose [7], facilitating the reversal of glucotoxicity, low carbohydrate diets are now recommended for disease control [10, 11].

In cases of hypoglycaemia, the owner can administer dextrose gels (Hypo-stop gel) or honey, jams or syrups to the mucous membranes of the mouth. This should only be recommended on advice from the veterinary surgeon once the owner has contacted the veterinary practice or the blood glucose level has been measured. Use of an at-home glucometer can be exceptionally useful, but obtaining sufficient blood for a test during a hypoglycaemic episode can be very difficult. This is due to a constriction of the peripheral blood supply, and in more severe cases, shaking or convulsions. Depending on glycaemic control, smaller frequent meals may prove to be more beneficial in obtaining control [8]. The use of continuous glucose monitoring (CGM) devices can give a fuller picture of the effect of the diet and frequency of eating for the clinician to make informed decisions [9].

Feeding an Obese Diabetic Cat

A controlled weight loss programme is required in these cases. Predisposition to hepatic lipidosis during rapid weight loss is of concern in cats and needs to be avoided with careful weight loss monitoring. Once an ideal body condition score has been achieved in these animals, and glucose levels remain stable, these animals must continue to receive regular clinical examinations, including weighing and fructosamine levels. Use of a higher-fat and -protein, decreased carbohydrate diet has proved to be very useful in these cases for steady weight loss.

The choice of diet will also depend on any secondary medical conditions. Renal dysfunction is commonly experienced when there has been a persistent hyperglycaemia. A low-phosphate diet would be a more preferable choice, but care should be taken, as these diets have higher carbohydrate content due to a restriction in protein levels. Weight loss if overweight or obese in patients with renal disease is not advised due to cachexia in renal disease as the disease progresses. If there is concurrent DM, recommendations need to be individualised to the patient.

Feeding a Diabetic Dog

On diagnosis of DM, a diet high in simple sugars should be avoided, as should semi-moist diets. These diets have a hyperglycaemic effect due to the increased levels of simple carbohydrates and other ingredients used as humectants (e.g. propylene glycol). Cost does play a deciding factor in choosing a diet for a diabetic patient. As does whether or not the animal eats the food. Diets that have a moderate fibre level with low simple sugars are exceptionally useful in aiding stabilisation of glucose control in dogs, but if the dog is unwilling to consume adequate amounts, this can be detrimental to the animal. An underweight animal will need a modified diet to gain weight, but this can only be achieved with insulin therapy.

Administration of exogenous insulin needs to be coordinated with times of feeding. Insulin regimes, whether insulin is being administered once or twice daily, will have a large effect on the quantities being fed at each mealtime. If injected once daily, half the food should be fed at the time of injection, the remainder eight to ten hours later. Twice daily injections require meals containing half the daily calorific intake at the same time as insulin administration. The owner needs to be aware of the detrimental effects of feeding snacks and treats between meals. Milk should also be avoided due to the calorific intake.

HYPERTHYROIDISM

Hyperthyroidism is more commonly observed in senior cats, caused by an overproduction of thyroid hormones (T3 and T4). The increase in these hormones forces the body's metabolism into overdrive, commonly resulting in weight loss, increased appetite, hyperactivity and increased thirst/urination (Figure 13.1).

Many of the observed clinical signs are gastrointestinal, and nutrition can help with these elements. As the demographic of hyperthyroid cats is in the older age range, their ability for assimilation of nutrients is decreased, and the use of a highly digestible diet (like a gastrointestinal diet) can be beneficial.

Nutritional Management of Hyperthyroidism

The endocrine disorder itself may also be managed through a diet devoid of iodine. As T3 and T4 require iodine to be produced, a relative deficiency in iodine will cause a reduction in the production of these hormones. The animal's intake of iodine needs to be closely monitored; with water sources also containing iodine, it can be difficult to control if the cat has access to the outside environment.

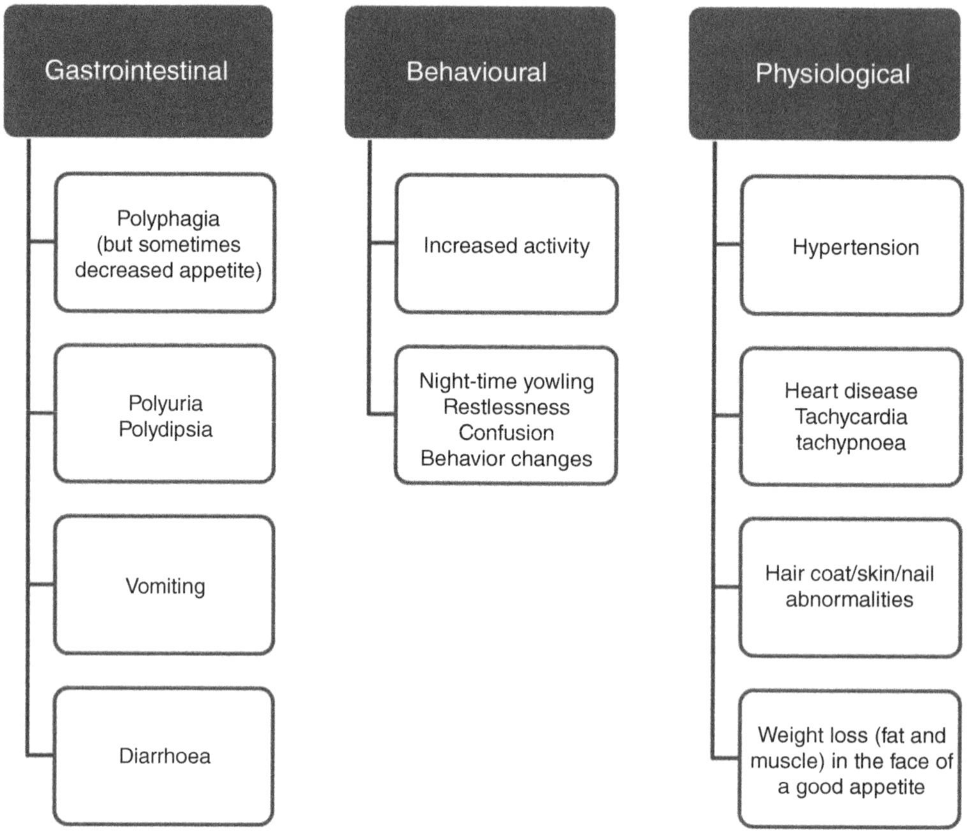

FIGURE 13.1 Clinical signs associated with hyperthyroidism in cats.

These diets can successfully manage hyperthyroidism, but as soon as another diet/food is fed to the animal, it will become hyperthyroid again.

HYPOTHYROIDISM

Hypothyroidism in dogs is a common disorder occurring when the thyroid gland produces insufficient thyroid hormones (T3 and T4), causing a significantly slowed metabolism. This underactive state usually affects middle-aged dogs, often leading to symptoms like weight gain, lethargy, cold intolerance, hair loss and poor skin/coat quality.

Nutritional interventions are surrounding helping to maintain an ideal body condition score. As these animals have a decrease in metabolism, diets that incorporate elements of nutrigenomics can be useful.

HYPERADRENOCORTICISM (HAC)

HAC or Cushing's syndrome is when the body produces too much cortisol.

Many of these animals also exhibit comorbidities such as pancreatitis, diabetes, urinary tract infections, hypertension and poor wound healing. Where comorbidities exist, nutritional interventions might be guided by these requirements (Figure 13.2).

There is no clear set of serum biochemistry results that point to Cushing's (Figure 13.3). The elevation of serum cortisol during dynamic testing is required. Dynamic testing includes the Low Dose Dexamethasone Suppression Test (LDDST) and the Adrenocorticotropic Hormone (ACTH) Stimulation Test.

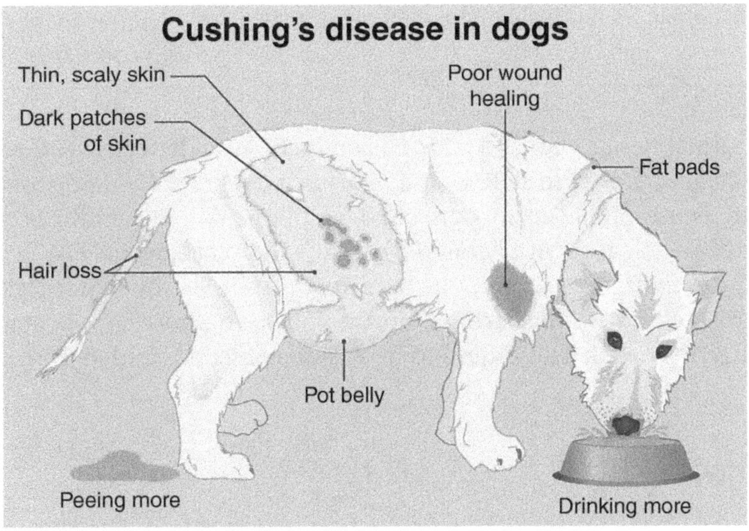

FIGURE 13.2 Clinical signs associated with hyperadrenocorticism (HAC).

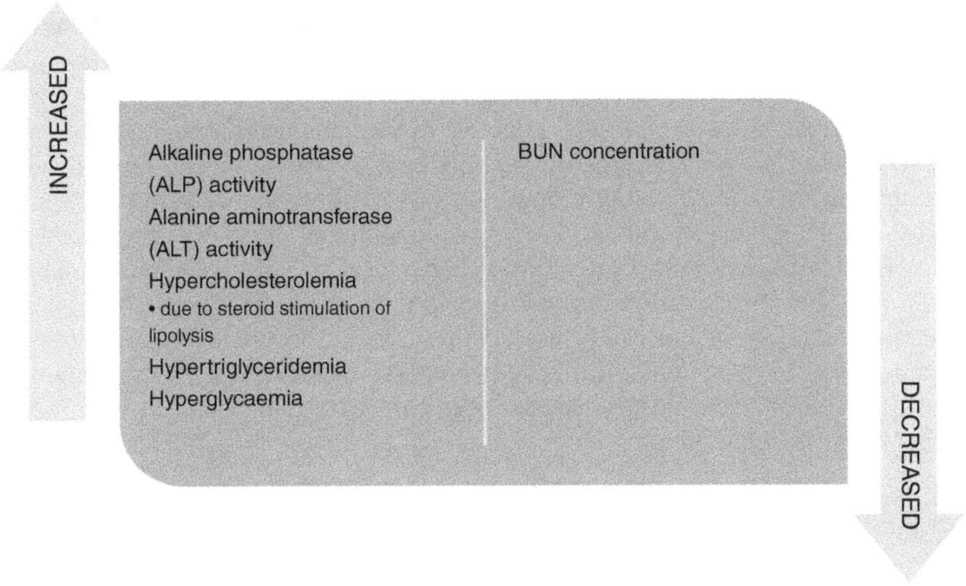

FIGURE 13.3 Serum biochemical abnormalities associated with hypercortisolaemia.

TABLE 13.1 Clinical signs often associated with hypoadrenocorticism (Addison's disease).

	Almost all cases	Common	Less common
Clinical history	Inappetence Lethargy	Weakness Vomiting	Diarrhoea Weight loss Shivering/muscle stiffness Polyuria Polydipsia
Physical examination	Depression Weakness	Dehydration	Bradycardia Hypothermia

CBC abnormalities are nonspecific and can include evidence of RBC regeneration (erythrocytosis and nucleated RBCs) and a stress leukogram (leukocytosis characterised by mature neutrophilia, eosinopenia and lymphopenia). Basophilia is occasionally evident. There is no clear set of haematology that will point towards HAC.

Due to these changes in serum biochemistry, especially the hypertriglyceridemia and hyperglycaemia, diets that are low in fat and have a low simple sugar (glycaemic index) are advocated. These tend to be the diets recommended for animals with pancreatitis.

Hypoadrenocorticism (Addison's Disease)

Addison's disease can be difficult to diagnose due to the waxing and waning of clinical signs and symptoms (Table 13.1).

In unstable or untreated Addison's patients, an Addisonian crisis can occur, which will result in hyponatraemia, hyperkalaemia and hypoglycaemia. This is due to a consequence of loss of sodium and chloride ions into the urine. Sodium loss leads to extracellular fluid (ECF) volume depletion and often profound dehydration if fluid intake is inadequate. Replacement of this deficit in fluids and electrolytes is required.

These losses, however, can be ongoing during management, and therefore, to monitor the efficacy of treatment, electrolytes are measured. The normal serum sodium:potassium (Na^+:K^+) ratio in dogs and cats lies between 27:1 and 40:1. A low ratio (below 27:1) can be a valuable clue to the possibility of primary hypoadrenocorticism, especially if the ratio is greatly diminished. Dose rates of medications are based on Na/K ratios. Electrolyte monitoring is needed to taper the dose rates.

Nutritional interventions can be used in these cases. Sodium levels are key. Serum sodium levels need to be kept within the reference range. Trials with supplementing sodium in the diet might be needed. Extreme care with diets that are restricted in sodium (e.g. some renal diets).

REFERENCES

1. Michel, K.E. (2005). Nutritional management of endocrine disease. In: *Textbook of Veterinary Internal Medicine*, 6e, vol. 1 (ed. S.J. Ettinger and E.C. Feldman). Missouri: Elsevier Science.

2. Stogale, L. (1986). Definition of diabetes mellitus. *Cornell Vet.* 76: 156.
3. Mazzaferro, E.M., Greco, D.S., Turner, A.S., and Fettman, M.J. (2003). Treatment of feline diabetes mellitus using an a-glucosidase inhibitor and a low carbohydrate diet. *J. Feline Med. Surg.* 5 (3): 183–189.
4. Hadd, M.J., Bienhoff, S.E., Little, S.E. et al. (2023). Safety and effectiveness of the sodium-glucose cotransporter inhibitor bexagliflozin in cats newly diagnosed with diabetes mellitus. *J. Vet. Int. Med.* 37 (3): 915.
5. Gostelow, R., Forcada, Y., Graves, T. et al. (2014). Systematic review of feline diabetic remission: separating fact from opinion. *Vet. J.* 202 (1): 208–221.
6. Link, K.R., Allio, I., Rand, J.S., and Eppler, E. (2013). The effect of experimentally induced chronic hyperglycaemia on serum and pancreatic insulin, pancreatic islet IGF-I and plasma and urinary ketones in the domestic cat (*Felis felis*). *Gen. Comp. Endocrinol.* 188: 269–281.
7. Singh, R., Rand, J.S., Coradini, M., and Morton, J.M. (2015). Effect of acarbose on postprandial blood glucose concentrations in healthy cats fed low and high carbohydrate diets. *J. Feline Med. Surg.* 17 (1): 848–857.
8. Behrend, E., Holford, A., Lathan, P. et al. (2018). 2018 AAHA diabetes management guidelines for dogs and cats. *J. Am. Anim. Hosp. Assoc.* 54 (1): 1–21.
9. Gottlieb, S. and Rand, J. (2018). Managing feline diabetes: current perspectives. *Vet. Med. (Auckl.)* 9: 33–42.
10. Bennett, N., Greco, D.S., Peterson, M.E. et al. (2006). Comparison of a low carbohydrate–low fiber diet and a moderate carbohydrate–high fiber diet in the management of feline diabetes mellitus. *J. Feline Med. Surg.* https://doi.org/10.1016/j.jfms.2005.08.004.
11. Frank, G., Anderson, W., Pazak, H. et al. (2001). Use of a high-protein food in the management of feline diabetes mellitus. *Vet. Therapeu.* 2: 238–246.

CHAPTER 14

Gastrointestinal Disease

CLINICAL NUTRITION

The clinical nutrition for each specific gastrointestinal (GI) issue is discussed separately below.

Adverse Reactions to Food – GI

Food allergies (food hypersensitivity) have an immunological basis and cause an adverse reaction to food or food additives. Food intolerances are non-immunological, where abnormal physiological responses to food or a food additive occur [1]. Specific food additives, which are known to cause problems, include onions and propylene glycol, which can cause haematological abnormalities in cats. Lactose intolerance is a relatively common metabolic adverse reaction in dogs and cats. Diarrhoea can develop when given cows' or even goats' milk, due to the lactose content being higher than that of bitch's or queen's milk. Gluten-sensitive enteropathy has been well documented in Irish Setters.

The role of elimination food trials often alleviates the signs of inflammatory bowel disease (IBD), which does seem to imply that food allergies or food intolerances play a role in this syndrome [1]. For further information on clinical nutrition for patients suffering from adverse food reactions, see the Chapter 12.

Acute Gastroenteritis and Vomiting, or Small Bowel Diarrhoea

Acute vomiting and diarrhoea are the most common reasons animals are presented to the veterinary practice. The definition of diarrhoea is an abnormal increase in frequency, water content or volume of faeces. This can result in the reduced absorption of nutrients and the loss of water, electrolytes and water-soluble nutrients, which can lead to dehydration and acidosis. Acute diarrhoea can be subdivided into four categories, described in detail in Table 14.1.

TABLE 14.1 Classification and pathophysiology of diarrhoea.

Classification of acute diarrhoea	Pathophysiology	Commonly causes
Osmotic	Excess water-soluble molecules in the intestinal lumen result in osmotic retention of water. D+ occurs when the fluid volume overwhelms the absorptive capacity of the small intestine and colon.	Sudden dietary change, malabsorption.
Permeability (exudative)	Inflammation in the intestine can stimulate increased secretion of fluid and electrolytes and impair absorption.	Permeability can be affected by ulceration, especially in cases of neoplastic disease. Where severe damage is present, serum protein and blood loss can also occur. Portal hypertension can also result in exudation of fluid into the intestinal lumen.
Secretory	When the absorptive capacities of the small intestine and colon are exceeded. Resulting D^+ can be severe and does not usually resolve with fasting.	Toxin release by enteric infectious agents (e.g. *Giardia* spp. and *Escherichia coli*).
Dysmotility	D+ can result in secondary alterations in motility, usually reduced intestinal motility.	Ileus and abnormal dilation of the intestine can be physical, neuromuscular, metabolic or functional abnormalities and can further promote D^+ as stasis allows for bacterial fermentation.

Adapted from Ref. [2].

The cause of acute diarrhoea and vomiting is most commonly due to irritation of the gut mucosa by toxins, infections and dysbiosis. The clinical symptoms of vomiting and diarrhoea are a response to remove the causal agent from the GI tract. In some cases, abrupt changes to the animal's diet can induce these symptoms as a causal factor in dysbiosis. In these cases, it is wise to stop feeding the new diet and, once the animal has returned to full health on the previous diet, initiate a slower transitional change to the new one. Support of the GI biome might also be required during the transition period. It is important to differentiate between small and large intestinal diarrhoea, as management can vary. (Table 14.2).

When using nutritional management with these cases, starting the animal on a highly digestible diet is recommended and feeding small, frequent meals. Specific veterinary clinical diets do offer a more balanced and complete nutritional meal than home-cooked ones, as they will also cater for losses of electrolytes and vitamins lost through vomiting and diarrhoea.

Nutraceuticals are frequently used in these cases and can be provided with the addition of pro-, pre- and postbiotics, absorbents and glutamine. The purpose

TABLE 14.2 Differences between small and large intestinal diarrhoea in the cat and dog.

Clinical symptom	Small intestinal diarrhoea	Large intestinal diarrhoea
Blood in faeces	Melena	Haematochezia
Frequency of defecation	Mild increase (<3 × day)	Markedly increased (>3 × day)
Faecal volume	Large quantities	Small quantities
Faecal quality	Loose, watery, 'cow-pie'	Loose to semi-formed, 'jelly-like'
Urgency	Usually absent	Often present
Tenesmus	Rare	Common
Faecal mucus	Rare	Common
Dyschezia	Absent	May be present
Vomiting	May be present	May be present
Weight loss	Common	Rare
Flatus/borborygmi	May be present	May be present

of absorbents is to bind bacteria and toxins, to protect the intestinal mucosa, and potentially for an antisecretory effect [2]. Kaolin has been traditionally used, but montmorillonite has been reported to be twenty times more effective than kaolin at absorbing pathogens [2].

FEEDING THROUGH

In human medicine, there is a continuing body of evidence indicating that 'feeding through' diarrhoea with an appropriate diet can be beneficial. Comparisons can be difficult, as many cases of diarrhoea in man tend to be secretory, whereas osmotic diarrhoea is more common in dogs and cats [3]. The advantages of feeding through include maintaining mucosal health, reducing the risk of bacterial translocation, and aiding in the 'flushing out' of the causal factor. Feeding through should not be used in animals that are vomiting or severely dehydrated. With animals where the GI tract is not functioning, the animal's nutritional requirements should be met through parenteral nutrition. The obvious disadvantage is the risk of 'accidents' in the house and the increase in faecal volume. Access to water must be maintained at all times and monitored. The use of oral rehydration solutions containing carbohydrates, peptides and electrolytes can be advocated in these cases. When using this method, feeding a diet which won't cause an inflammatory reaction in the future can be important. Dietary antigens can cross the compromised GI mucosa and set up a hypersensitivity reaction. Use of a novel protein and/or carbohydrate source can be recommended in chronic cases. Once the animal is well and transferred to its original diet, it is unlikely to have any reactions to the original protein source.

Anal Glands and Impactions

Anal gland impactions can occur when the dog or cat's diet is low or restricted in fibre. The inclusion of fibre into the diet acts as a bulking agent and allows a constant pressure on the glands at defecation. Decreasing the risk of the glands becoming full. Glands that become overfilled have a higher risk of becoming infected and/or impacted. Dietary management of these cases is necessary, and the inclusion of fibre into the diet is warranted. This can be achieved by feeding a higher fibre diet or by the addition of fibre-containing pellets. The anal glands do have their own biome, and a dysbiosis of the gland can also be an issue. The role of the synbiotic trio can be of use in this correction back to a balanced biome.

Where anal gland surgery has been performed, the use of a low-residue (low fibre) diet is advocated to remove pressure from suture lines. Once the incision wounds have healed, a nutritional assessment is required to give an updated nutritional recommendation.

Borborygmus and Flatulence

Borborygmus and flatulence are very common occurrences in many animals. This can be due to the diet, or the rapid consumption of the diet, which leads to aerophagia or the GI biome and its response to the diet. A slow dietary change can be recommended in some of these cases. For dogs that are aerophagic, any feeding method that slows down consumption or reduces the swallowing of air needs to be advocated. This can take time to determine the most positive method. The diet can be spread out on a flat surface, slow feeders, scatter feeding, fed little and often, and adding water to the diet can all aid in increasing consumption time.

Dietary management is concerned with decreasing the intestinal gas production by bacterial fermentation of undigested foods. Commercial products are available for reducing flatulence. These products can contain α-galactosidase and reduce flatulence by improving the digestion of nonabsorbable carbohydrates [4]. Diets that increase intestinal microbial activity have been attributed to increased levels of flatulence, as have vitamin and mineral supplements, due to the increased levels of fermentation [4]. Other veterinary medicines can contain antacids, aluminium hydroxide and magnesium trisilicate as well as copper complexes of chlorophyllins. Clinical trials have demonstrated efficacy in reducing wind and smells and relieving indigestion and gastric upset in the dog. The local antacid effect in the stomach promotes coalescence and removal of trapped gases from the gut contents, thereby limiting their passage through into the later stages of the GI tract. It should also be noted that in certain breeds (mainly Brachycephalics), aerophagia is common due to the conformation of the face, but also note that the prevalence of regurgitation is higher in these breeds due to the positive pressure changes.

Chronic Diarrhoea

Chronic diarrhoea can be a range of clinical signs from a vast number of different problems. It is essential to determine the underlying cause so that specific treatments for each case can be initiated. Dietary management plays an important role in the diagnosis and the long-term management of these cases, as relapses can be frequent. As each case is different, there is no one specific diet aimed at animals suffering from chronic diarrhoea. Recommendations of low-fat, single (sometimes novel) protein diets that are highly digestible are given. Yet in some cases, diets that have a high-fibre content are the diet of choice in resolving the clinical symptoms.

INFLAMMATORY BOWEL DISEASE (IBD)

The management of IBD involves the combined use of anti-inflammatory medication alongside the use of a single novel protein diet. A full dietary history is required to ascertain what protein sources the animal has been exposed to. Diets, which contain novel protein sources such as venison or duck, have proved to be beneficial, as initially, lamb was used as a novel protein source. Subsequently, many life-stage diets now include lamb and are marketed to animals with sensitive stomachs. When using an elimination diet, it is important to challenge the system to see if the original diet was the initial cause. See Chapter 12 for further details.

The use of fermentable fibre in these cases should not be underestimated. Colonic bacteria easily digest fermentable fibres, which in turn produce butyrate, a short-chain fatty acid. Butyrate is the primary energy source for colonocytes and thus helps to maintain gut health. Other SCFAs are also produced, which reduce the colonic pH and thus reduce the risk of pathogenic bacteria colonising the area. As the body absorbs the SCFA, there is an increase in the absorption of electrolytes and water from the colon. The role of the gut biome in IBS is important; studies have shown that recurrent use of some antimicrobials, like metronidazole, will have a ninefold increase of IBS in later life. The mechanisms of the antimicrobials' impact on the biome do require further investigation.

When feeding an animal with IBD, the nutritional goal is to provide adequate nutrient intake to meet the requirements of the individual but also to compensate for ongoing losses through the GI tract.

PROTEIN-LOSING ENTEROPATHY (PLE) AND LYMPHANGIECTASIA

Lymphangiectasia is characterised by abnormalities of the intestinal lymphatic system. The condition can be a primary defect of the lymphatic system or secondary as a consequence of severe intestinal infiltrative disease (e.g. IBD, lymphosarcoma) [5]. Lymphangiectasia is the most common cause of PLE in dogs and cats. Not all animals present with the clinical symptom of diarrhoea but often present with progressive weight loss, even with a good calorific consumption. The leaky intestinal lymphatics result in hypoalbuminemia and loss of colloidal oncotic pressure.

When feeding animals with PLE, the key is to control dietary fat levels. Long-chain triglycerides provide a major stimulus for intestinal lymph flow; the protein content of the lymph tends to increase with the dietary fat content. Limiting dietary fat content will reduce the lymphatic flow, reduce lacteal and lymphatic distension and thus minimise protein losses [5]. Dietary fat levels of <10% DMB for dogs and <15% DMB for cats are recommended [5]. The protein levels of the diet are important; feeding a high-protein diet is often unsuccessful. The cause of the PLE is important, as in cases where severe IBD is the underlying cause, care should be given when selecting a protein source. Protein levels should be of a high biological value, and levels in excess of 25% DMB for dogs and in excess of 35% DMB in cats have been recommended [5].

COLITIS

Colitis is the most common cause of diarrhoea in dogs and cats. Colitis (inflammation of the colon) is characterised by the presence of mucus covering the faeces and/or fresh blood. There are many causes of colitis, including stress. Many dogs have colitis when being hospitalised at veterinary practices due to stress levels. Management of mild cases is through nutritional changes, though in chronic or severe cases, medical treatment may be required alongside dietary management. Modifications to the diet include:

- High-fibre diets that normalise the transit time and bind faecal water. Fibre also acts as a prebiotic, aiding the strains and populations of gut bacteria.
- Low-fibre, highly digestible diets will aid in reducing the quantity of undigested food entering the colon.
- Hypoallergenic diets can also be used when an intolerance or hypersensitivity is present.

When the initiating cause of the colitis is unknown, dietary modifications can be very much trial and error, as the first two (high-fibre and low-fibre) do contraindicate each other. This should be relayed to owners so that they have a better understanding of the problem and that they do not get frustrated with dietary management. It is also recommended to advise owners that colitis is normally seen spasmodically, with intervals of normality between bouts.

CONSTIPATION/MEGACOLON

Constipation in animals can be due to a clinical symptom of systemic disease, a response to diet or nutrient changes, or as a consequence of damage to the pelvis. Constipation is characterised by the absence, infrequency or difficulty in defecation associated with retention of faeces within the colon and rectum [4]. The treatment and preventative management of constipation do differ. The addition of fibre to the diet, whilst the animal is constipated, can lead to compounding the initial problem. Treatments can include enemas and laxatives. To prevent the recurrence of constipation, a full history is required to identify the causal factor or factors. The water and fibre consumption of the animal needs to be ascertained. Maintenance of normal hydration levels is required; intake of water should be 40 to 60 ml/kg body weight per day. Recommendations to increase water intake in animals are detailed in the appendix. Fibre intake can be estimated from the analysis of the pet food label.

Increasing the fibre content of the diet can improve constipation dramatically. Increasing the amounts of fibre in the diet can aid in increasing the water content of the faeces, intestinal transit rates and colonic motility. When increasing the dietary fibre content of the diet, it should be remembered that fermentable and non-fermentable fibres should be included. The palatability of high-fibre foods can be decreased, and the transition to a fibre-enhanced veterinary therapeutic diet can be difficult. In some cases, remaining on the original diet and adding a fibre source can be utilised. Some animals can suffer side effects when changed to a high-fibre diet if the transition is done too quickly. Flatulence and abdominal cramping are common side effects of the addition of fermentable fibres. Some animals can develop megacolon or constipation when fed a moderate to high fibre (>15% DM crude fibre). The transition to these diets should be made in increments of increasing fibre content. If such side effects do occur, then it is recommended that the fibre content be decreased by 5% DMB, and the animal is to be reassessed. Up to 10% fibre can be added to the diet without compromising its overall nutrient balance. Titration of the dietary fibre content of the diet can be achieved by the use of food combinations with diets of varying crude fibre content.

In situations of severe constipation or megacolon where colonic motility is not present, the use of high-fibre diets is not recommended. In these cases, a highly digestible diet (dry matter digestibility >90%) is the diet of choice. This will have an exceptionally low residue whilst still providing adequate calories. The faecal production is minimal enough that removal of the faeces can be achieved via enemas once or twice weekly.

The use of medical therapies in aid of constipation is an important adjunct to dietary management and is suitable for mild to moderate constipation. Laxatives, lactulose and sorbitol are poorly absorbed carbohydrates and prove to be very useful. These sugars are hydrolysed to fatty acids by the colonic microflora, where they exert osmotic pressure and draw fluid into the colonic lumen. Colonic motility modifiers such as cisapride are also of use, especially in rabbits. The dose rate is 0.25 mg/kg bwt, t.i.d. to q.i.d. in dogs and cats [1]. Treatment of constipation and megacolon in animals is very much case-specific and can be dependent on the initiating case.

GASTRIC DILATION-VOLVULUS

Gastric dilation-volvulus (GDV), or bloat, is thought to be the final common pathway of a variety of problems in certain predisposed large-breed dogs, though GD and GDVs can occur in any species or breed [1]. Gastric dilation is defined as the distension of the stomach with a mixture of air, food and fluid. GDV occurs when the rotation of the stomach on its mesenteric axis happens. This entraps the gastric contents, whilst also compromising the vascular supply to the stomach, spleen and pancreas. Breeds which are predisposed are large, deep-chested dogs, including Irish Setters, Great Danes, Standard Poodles, Doberman Pinschers, German Shepherds and Saint Bernards. Dogs with a BCS of ⊆2/5 are also considered a risk factor for GDV. Males are twice as likely as females to develop GDV. Also, if a parent has experienced GDV the risk is greatly increased. This can be as high as 63% greater risk if a first-degree relative has suffered from GDV [6].

Diet can play some role in susceptible animals, but no diet-related cause has been clearly identified [1]. Several dietary risk factors have been identified, and these include:

- Feeding only one meal per day.
- Postprandial exercise, especially vigorous exercise. Recommendations include avoiding exercise one hour pre- and two hours postprandial. Gentle exercise has been shown to improve GI functioning.
- Rapid consumption of food, leading to aerophagia. Slowing of food intake can be aided by placing the food on a flat baking tray or spreading the dry food out on the floor (scatter feeding) and using puzzle feeders and slow feeders.
- Food particle/kibble diameter of less than 30 mm.
- Consumption of large volumes of water. Water needs to be available at all times so that the animal can drink little and often. If large consumptions of water do occur postprandially, this can be problematic. Limiting water consumption in this period can help, also mixing wet and dry diets.
- Episodes of overeating.
- Sudden changes in diets. All dietary transitions should be performed slowly; see Chapter 12 for details.

The consumption of dry diets has been blamed in the past for being a predisposing factor for GDVs; epidemiological studies have shown this to be an incorrect assumption [5]. Other dogs that seem to be predisposed to GDV are those which tend to be nervous and anxious. These dogs should always be fed in a situation that is best suited for them.

Feeding a Dog Predisposed to GDV

As there are no specific nutritional factors that have been established for GD or GDV, it is difficult to advise on a specific dietary regime for these animals. The diet fed needs to provide all the adequate nutrients and energy requirements for that particular life stage and BCS. The daily management of the dog is important and includes dividing the diet into small, frequent meals; feeding in a manner that reduces any aerophagia; avoiding exercise around the times of feeding; decreasing competitive feeding; feeding a mixture of moist and dry diets; increasing the time it takes for the dog to consume the diet; and avoiding excess water consumption postprandially.

Owners should always be advised of the symptoms of GD or GDV in all breeds that are predisposed. In veterinary practices, it is advisable to inform clients of this when they initially present their puppies at puppy clinics or at the initial vaccinations.

HAIRBALLS IN CATS AND RABBITS

Hairballs are a common occurrence in cats, though cats with longer, thicker coats or those with fastidious grooming behaviour do tend to suffer more. Hairballs do not usually cause clinical disease, though vomiting can be a nuisance or even distressing for owners. Laxatives and lubricants can be utilised, either with or without specialised diets, for the routine management of hairballs. The use of lubricants and laxatives should be limited due to the interference with normal digestion and absorption of nutrients.

Hairballs are loose accumulations of hair and mucus which form in the digestive tract. In some cases, the hair and mucus can form with other materials to form trichobezoars, which are much harder. Trichobezoars form within the stomach or intestines and are less common in cats but are a common cause of anorexia in rabbits. If the trichobezoars become large enough, obstruction of the pylorus or intestines can occur. Hairballs are a common finding in rabbits due to their inability to vomit and should be considered even in short-haired animals which present with anorexia. Often, on palpation of the stomach, a large doughy mass can be felt. Treatment for trichobezoars is based on breaking down the proteinaceous matrix that binds them together. Large trichobezoars must be removed via surgery or endoscopy [1]. If left, obstructions and ileus can occur. Survival after surgery of the digestive tract, particularly gastrotomy, is reportedly low in rabbits [7]. Hairballs in rabbits can be prevented by feeding a diet with adequate dietary fibre (>14% DM crude fibre), minimising stress and boredom, encouraging movement and thus transit times of the GIT, and grooming the animal frequently [6].

A common treatment for hairballs is pineapple juice and papaya juice, the supposed active ingredients being the enzyme bromelain (in pineapple juice) and papain (in papaya juice). There is no evidence to support this, and in truth, the enzymes bromelain and papain are incapable of dissolving keratin, the main protein component of hair [7, 8]. Simple sugars in the fruit juices may promote overgrowth of *Clostridium* spp. [8] (Figure 14.1).

Stress

⇓

Decreased GI motility

⇓

Inappetence

⇓

Imbalance of caecal flora/dehydration

⇓

Overgrowth of yeast and *Clostridium* spp.

⇓

Gas and toxin production by *Clostridium* spp.

⇓

GIT pain.

⇓

Further decrease in motility/persistent anorexia.

⇓

Liver damage due to toxins/lipidosis

⇓

Death.

FIGURE 14.1 Downward cascade of factors relating to ileus. Adapted from Ref. [8].

REFERENCES

1. Buffington, T., Holloway, C., and Abood, S. (2004). *Manual of Veterinary Dietetics*. Missouri: Elsevier Saunders.
2. Battersby, I. and Harvey, A. (2006). Differential diagnosis and treatment of acute diarrhoea in the dog and cat. *In Pract.* 28: 480–488.
3. McCann, T. and Simpson, J.W. (2006). Approach to the management of diarrhoea. *Companion Animal* 11 (6): 30–37.
4. Davenport, D.J., Remillard, R.L., Simpson, K.W., and Pidgeon, G.L. (2000). Gastrointestinal and exocrine pancreatic disease. In: *Small Animal Clinical Nutrition*, 4e (ed. M.S. Hand, C.D. Thatcher, R.L. Remillard, and P. Roudebush), 725–810. Missouri: Mark Morris Institute.
5. Elwood, C.M. (1998). Risk factors for gastric dilation in Irish setter dogs. *J. Small Anim. Pract.* 39: 185–190.
6. Ragni, R.A. (2005). GDV: preventing the nightmare is best. *Veterinary Times* (31st October), pp. 6–7.
7. Brewer, N.R. and Cruise, L.J. (1994). Physiology. In: *The Biology of the Laboratory Rabbit* (ed. P.J. Manning, D.H. Ringer, and C.E. Newcomer), 65. San Diego: Academic Press.
8. Watson, P.J. (2005). Managing canine pancreatitis. *BSAVA Congress 2005 Scientific Proceedings*, 97–99.

CHAPTER 15

Hepatic Disorders

HEPATOBILIARY DISEASE

The liver is critical in maintaining homeostasis and removing waste products that have accumulated within the body. The liver is essential in producing proteins and the deamination of excessive, unneeded proteins. Understanding the functioning of the organ is essential in designing a diet relating to the clinical symptoms that the animal is exhibiting.

Key Liver Functions

- Detoxification: Filters blood, removes toxins, bacteria and breaks down drugs and alcohol.
- Digestion and metabolism: Produces bile to break down fats and metabolises carbohydrates, proteins and fats.
- Storage: Stores glucose as glycogen, along with vitamins (A, D, E, K and B12) and iron.
- Protein synthesis: Produces essential proteins for blood plasma, including albumin and blood-clotting factors.

The liver can be damaged in several different ways, from infection and hepatic encephalopathy (HE) as an adjunct to medical therapies and from toxins. Congenital abnormalities, such as portalsystemic shunts (PSS), will also affect how the liver functions (Figure 15.1). Analysis of laboratory results and other diagnostic means will enable the practitioner to identify where the damage is occurring within the liver. Delayed recovery from general anaesthesia may be the first indication of compromised liver function (Box 15.1).

The nutritional management of hepatobiliary disease is usually directed at clinical manifestations of the disease rather than the specific cause itself.

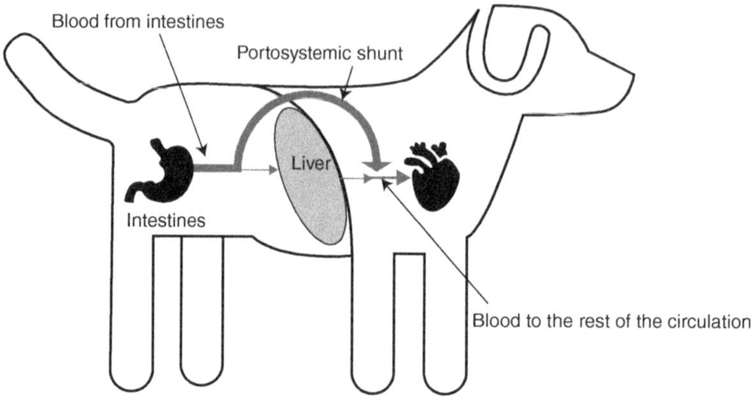

FIGURE 15.1 Diagrammatic representation of a portalsystemic shunt.

Box 15.1 Possible causes of hepatic issues

Infectious – Leptospirosis, ascending biliary infections and septicaemia
Inflammatory – Immune-mediated, idiopathic
Metabolic (lipidosis) – Idiopathic, secondary to starvation
Toxic – Drugs, mushroom consumption
Idiopathic – Chronic active hepatitis

The aims of nutritional management are:

- Maintaining the normal metabolic processes.
- Avoiding toxic by-product accumulation.
- Correcting any electrolyte disturbances.
- Providing substrates that support hepatocellular regeneration and repair.

There is no one 'ideal' liver disease treatment or diet. The dietary needs of the patient require a good understanding of what you are trying to achieve and the individual animal's needs. Personalisation of nutrition needs to occur. A palatable, high-quality protein diet, supplemented with zinc, B vitamins and antioxidants, should be fed. Protein should not be restricted unless it is essential to control encephalopathy. Malnutrition is a very common feature of chronic hepatic disease, and correct nutrition for each patient is important to help regulate the hormonal milieu that occurs with hepatic injury.

CLINICAL NUTRITION

Protein

The maintenance of a positive nitrogen balance is important for the preservation of body condition and protein synthesis. Protein malnutrition is common in patients with chronic liver disease, where the clinical manifestations include weight loss, loss of muscle tissue and hypoalbuminaemia. Protein intake needs to be in a fine balance; in some dogs, the protein requirements may exceed those of normal maintenance requirements due to the increased protein turnover and the demands of hepatocellular regeneration. A moderate restriction of protein levels is not always recommended, and the quality (Biological Value) of the proteins should be increased. This is recommended as they fulfil the animal's needs with minimal production of nitrogenous waste. Studies have shown that in human patients with hepatic failure, the nitrogen balance can be improved if the diet is divided into small, frequent meals. However, in some animals where the liver struggles with the deamination of any excessive protein in the diet, it is important that the protein levels are controlled within the diet.

Dairy products (cottage cheese, milk) can be of benefit, this is due to the related to factors such as the relatively high ratio of carbohydrates to protein, their influence on intestinal transit and colonic pH, as well as the differing amino acid composition. Fibre of soya origin has been shown to provide an excellent source of dietary fibre that reduces ammonia production and absorption in the colon and assists ammonia elimination in the faeces.

One of the roles of the liver is a protein regulatory event, including degradation of the essential amino acids (including the aromatic amino acids [AAA], but not the branched-chain amino acids [BCAA]) and some of the nonessential amino acids. Dogs and other omnivores are able to down-regulate the activities of protein degradation when minimal dietary protein is consumed; cats are not able to do this. Plasma amino acid concentrations differ depending on the type of hepatic failure. In the normal healthy animal, AAA (i.e. tyrosine, phenylalanine and tryptophan) are effectively extracted from the portal circulation and metabolised by the liver. Reduced hepatic function is associated with an increase in circulating AAA. Conversely, the plasma concentrations of BCAA (i.e. leucine, isoleucine and valine) and most other amino acids are reduced due to an increased rate of metabolism by muscle and adipose tissue. The ratio between AAA and BCAA can be used to evaluate liver function. In healthy dogs, the ratio between BCAA and AAA ranges between 3.0 and 4.0. This ratio can be reduced to 1.0 or less in dogs with portosystemic vascular anomalies and chronic hepatitis. Other factors, such as increased levels of insulin, glucagon and catecholamines, are thought to contribute to the altered amino acid metabolism seen in these patients. Alterations in this ratio have also been implicated in the pathogenesis of HE. Hence, BCAA-enriched solutions have been used in human nutritional support for many years in those patients suffering from chronic hepatic disease and HE.

Carbohydrates and Fats

Nonprotein calories should come from highly digestible carbohydrate and fat sources. The fat level in the diet should not be restricted unless there is clinical evidence of steatorrhoea.

Vitamins and Minerals

The requirement of vitamins and minerals within the diet is dependent on the causal problem within the liver. Copper levels should be restricted due to accumulation within the liver, and this is discussed further below. Vitamins, which are produced within the liver, should be supplemented, as deficiencies are common, for example, a deficiency of zinc. The severity of liver disease does correlate with oxidative damage, antioxidants should also be supplemented.

COPPER-ASSOCIATED HEPATOTOXICOSIS IN DOGS

Bedlington terriers can often develop copper storage disease and subsequently hepatitis and cirrhosis. Copper-associated hepatotoxicosis is caused by an inherited autosomal recessive trait that results in impaired biliary excretion of copper. Statistics state that roughly 25% of Bedlington terriers are affected, with 50% being genetic carriers. Some other breeds have also been affected, namely the West Highland White Terriers and Doberman Pinschers. Thus, diets for these dogs do need to have a reduction in the copper levels. Supplements containing copper should also be avoided. Homemade diets should not contain liver, shellfish and organ meats, which are all high in copper content.

The role of copper in hepatic diseases in other breeds of dogs is less clear. There are theories that elevated hepatic copper concentrations precede liver damage, whereas others contend that the excess hepatic copper results from faulty copper excretion caused by chronic cholestasis. A third theory is that elevated levels are antecedent to the disease and are incidental to disease progression. Anti-inflammatory agents, such as prednisolone, can be beneficial in the management of chronic hepatitis in Bedlington Terriers and West Highland White Terriers.

The nutritional aims of managing patients with copper-associated hepatotoxicosis are:

- To decrease further absorption of copper from the gastrointestinal tract.
- To enhance copper excretion.

PORTALSYSTEMIC SHUNTS (PSS) AND HEPATIC ENCEPHALOPATHY (HE)

PSS are vascular communications between the portal and systemic venous systems. This communication allows access of portal blood to the systemic circulation without passing through the liver. Congenital PSS are most common and are inherited. They may either be intrahepatic (large breeds such as Irish wolfhound and Burmese Mountain Dog) or extrahepatic (medium and toy breeds, such as Yorkshire terrier, Cairn terrier and Dachshund). Stunted growth or failure to gain weight can occur in these animals. Acquired PSS forms in response to portal hypertension caused by fibrosis and chronic cirrhosis. As a result of inadequate hepatic clearance of toxins and altered liver function, HE can result. Ammonium urate and other purine uroliths can also occur due to the high urinary excretion of ammonia and uric acid.

Shunting results in nutritional depletion of the liver as well as failed delivery of substrates to the liver for degradation and metabolism. HE is a complex metabolic disorder, which is characterised by abnormal mental status.

The nutritional aims for managing patients with HE include:

- Reducing excessive dietary protein.
- Changing intestinal flora.
- Decreasing intestinal transit time, quickening the transit of the stool.

Soluble or fermentable fibre in the diet, such as cellulose and lactulose, aids animals suffering from liver dysfunction as it helps reduce the side effects of deamination of proteins. These are forms of prebiotics. Lactulose is a synthetic disaccharide that is hydrolysed into short-chain fatty acids in the colon. The change in the lumen pH traps the ammonia as ammonium ions, which are removed in the faeces. There is also the beneficial effect that colonic bacteria use the increasing nitrogen in reproduction and growth, whilst also inhibiting ammonia generation by colonic bacteria through a process known as catabolite repression (Figure 15.2).

Insoluble or non-fermentable fibre is also an important constituent in the diet of animals suffering from hepatic disease. Constipation is a predisposing factor for the development of encephalopathy since it increases the contact time for colonic bacteria to act on the faeces and produce ammonia.

Vitamins and Minerals

Vitamin E is a superb antioxidant and may be cytoprotective, especially in copper toxicity, due to the effects it has in protecting against lipid peroxidation. Vitamin K supplementation may become a necessity if clotting times are prolonged, especially before hepatic biopsies are taken. The vitamin K stores within the liver are eliminated

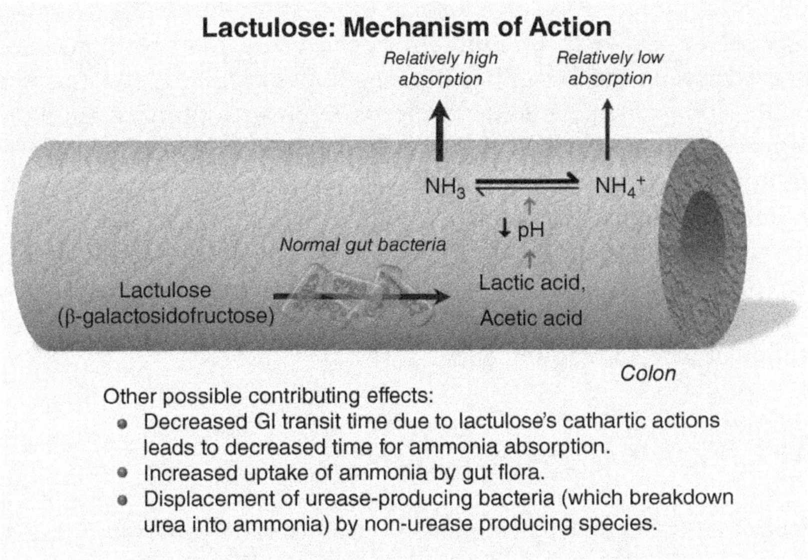

FIGURE 15.2 Diagrammatic representation of the action that lactulose plays to reduce the absorption of ammonia into the bloodstream.

and do become rapidly depleted, although the function for the synthesis of the prothrombin-complex clotting factors is always lost before the storage of vitamin K is depleted. The other fat-soluble vitamins A and D should not be supplemented, as vitamin A can cause hepatic damage and vitamin D can cause calcification within the tissues.

The level of calorific intake determines the requirements for the water-soluble vitamins. Thus, if anorexia is present, the requirement is low, though when nutrition intake increases, the water-soluble vitamins are required to replenish coenzymes involved in metabolic processes in the liver and other tissues. As with all animals suffering from polydipsia and polyuria, supplementation with B vitamins is required. Animals suffering from hepatic disease have been recommended to receive a double dose of B vitamins. Vitamin C should not be supplemented as it can increase the tissue damage associated with copper and iron disease.

Choline is essential in the packaging of very low-density lipoproteins (VLDL) in the liver and, therefore, the exportation of triglycerides. A choline deficiency with concurrent lipolysis may slow down VLDL export and promote hepatic lipid accumulation. Hepatic diets should contain supplementation of choline and carnitine, but the efficacy levels are unknown.

There are large amounts of supportive data that zinc deficiency is common in hepatic injury. This is due to a reduction in absorption and an increase in loss via the urine. Nutrition supplementation of the diet with zinc reduces encephalopathy; at an effective rate, the same as lactulose.

FEEDING A HEPATIC DIET

The dietary modifications aim to meet the animal's daily requirement for nutrients whilst reducing the metabolic demands placed upon the liver. The calorific needs of the liver should be met with non-protein calories, and the nutritional deficiencies which can occur due to the loss of hepatic function need to be met within the diet.

Frequent feeding of small meals is preferred to ensure optimal assimilation and to limit the entry of dietary protein into the colon. Other complications of liver disease include gastrointestinal ulceration and ascites. If ulceration is known to be present, the animal must not go without food.

Regular monitoring of the body condition score and muscle condition score needs to be undertaken. Any reduction in muscle mass needs to be addressed. Quantitative monitoring of blood plasma proteins can occur; albumin and globulin levels give a good reflection of protein requirements.

IDIOPATHIC FELINE HEPATIC LIPIDOSIS

The incidence rate of feline hepatic lipidosis is unfortunately increasing. Most of these cats are obese and usually present with a history of prolonged anorexia after a stressful event. Hepatic lipidosis is characterised by the accumulation of excess triglycerides in the hepatocytes, which results in cholestasis and hepatic dysfunction. This disease may be idiopathic or may develop secondary to some underlying medical problem. Hepatic lipidosis is more commonly seen in cats due to several special features, which make the cat less tolerant to periods of anorexia. Reasons for this include the cat's reduced ability to synthesise arginine being lower than that of other species. This specific amino acid is an intermediate of the urea cycle, in which ammonia is converted to urea. Its other role is in the production of apoproteins, which are incorporated into VLDL. VLDL transports triglycerides from the liver to adipose tissue. Any changes in the availability of arginine can result in hyperammonaemia, even when there is minimal hepatic dysfunction, and a disturbance to the transportation of triglycerides. Taurine is also required in VLDL production and the conjugation of bile acids. As taurine is also required in larger amounts in the cat, any deficiencies can result in VLDL disturbances. L-Carnitine is also essential in the transportation of long-chain fatty acids into the mitochondria. L-Carnitine is often supplemented into hepatic diets and obesity diets for this very reason, aiding in the mobilisation of circulating fats. If any of these supply chains become unbalanced, then hepatic lipidosis can occur. Since any disruption in hepatic lipid metabolism can cause lipidosis, it is unlikely that there is a common cause for all cases of feline hepatic lipidosis. Hypokalaemia is present in about 30% of cats with severe hepatic lipidosis; hence, electrolyte monitoring is important, as hypokalaemia can prolong anorexia and exacerbate the expression of HE (Figure 15.3).

Insulin resistance with subsequent glucose intolerance represents a key metabolic abnormality in all patients with chronic hepatic injury. This can be due to reduced insulin activity from depletion of insulin receptors on the target cells. Hence, many cats with hepatic lipidosis are hyperglycaemic. Reduced insulin activity results in activation of triacylglycerol lipase, with consequent hydrolysis of triglycerols. This results in the increased release of free fatty acids into the circulation from the adipose tissue.

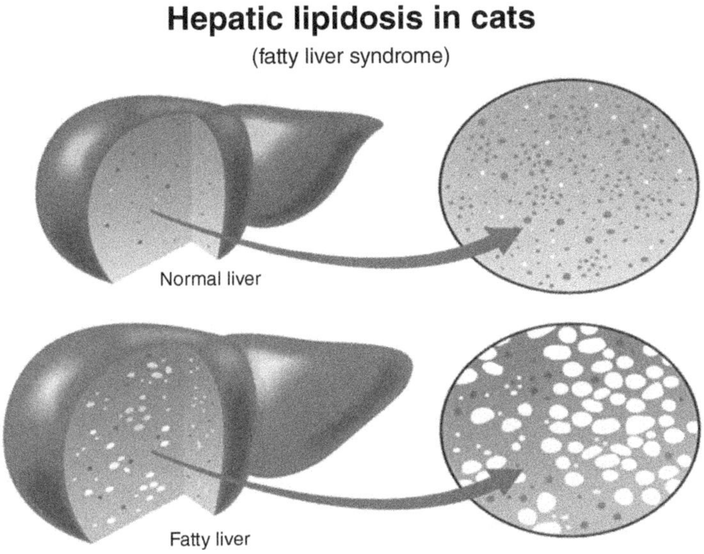

FIGURE 15.3 Diagrammatic representation of hepatic lipidosis in cats.

Treatment of Feline Hepatic Lipidosis

Nutrition plays a supportive role in the management of most hepatic diseases, but nutritional therapy is the primary treatment for feline idiopathic hepatic lipidosis. It is a condition that requires vigorous supportive care; this includes intravenous fluids and nutritional support. The provision of an adequate daily energy intake is the cornerstone of successful medical management. This can only truly be achieved through early tube feeding via a nasogastric tube. Force-feeding of the cat rarely meets the calorific needs of the cat. Food aversion is an exceptionally important component to be considered when tempting anorexic cats, hence why tube feeding is a more preferable method. Intravenous feeding (total parenteral feeding) is not recommended unless some enteral nutrition is also being concurrently provided. Parenteral feeding is associated with hepatic steatosis, villus atrophy, fluid and electrolyte imbalances, and an increased incidence of sepsis. This is due to enteral nutrition providing antigenic stimulation to the gut-associated lymphoid tissue (GALT) and stimulating secretion of IgA, which helps to maintain an intact gastrointestinal barrier, to prevent bacterial translocation. Other factors that need to be considered in these cases include:

- Correction of hypokalaemia. This can be achieved by potassium supplementation through intravenous fluids and oral, tube feeding methods.
- Correction of hyperglycaemia and the cell uptake of these calories. Carbohydrates should not replace dietary fat due to glucose intolerance.
- Dietary protein intake needs to be adapted to suit the individual patient. It is advised that the protein intake should not be reduced below 20% of calories from this source.
- When starting tube feeding, a balanced formulation sufficient to meet the cat's RER at its current weight is ideal. In grossly obese cats carrying 35% or more fat, they should be fed at a lower estimated optimal weight rather than their current weight.

It is important that, where cats have been anorexic, Refeeding syndrome can occur. Reinstating feeding needs to be done slowly over several days. See Chapter 9. Hydration and electrolyte levels need to be corrected before any nutrition can be administered.

SUPPLEMENTS

Nutraceuticals can be beneficial in some hepatic conditions; these include toxicities (pharmaceutical/plant), chronic active hepatitis, hepatic lipidosis, cholangitis, cholangiohepatitis, patients receiving drugs with hepatotoxic potential and patients with decreased hepatobiliary function. Both *S*-adenosylmethionine (SAMe) and the silymarin complexes have proven to be beneficial.

S-ADENOSYLMETHIONINE (SAMe)

Glutathione is a major antioxidant produced by the liver; its main function is to reduce oxidative damage to the hepatocytes by free radicals. When the liver is compromised, there is an increased production of free radicals, and the extent of the oxidative stress suffered by hepatocytes is increased. An increased supply of glutathione is required, as production is also decreased during hepatic disease. The supply of glutathione is via SAMe. SAMe initiates three major biochemical pathways: transmethylation, transsulfuration and aminopropylation, which all help promote liver health and preserve functioning liver tissue. SAMe is found endogenously (within the body), being synthesised by the body's cells, including hepatocytes. SAMe is derived from ATP and methionine, and it initiates biochemical pathways involved in critical functions such as detoxification, modulating steroid hormone effects, cellular function, and intracellular communication; regulating the NA/K ATPase pump; and protecting cellular DNA. SAMe also has other important roles, including cytoprotection, modulating inflammation, promoting cell replication, protein synthesis and improving hepatocellular function.

Milk Thistle

Milk thistle is an herb which contains an active antioxidant bioflavonoid complex known as silymarin. Silymarin stimulates the production of glutathione and glutathione peroxidase (also refer to 'Antioxidants' section in Chapter 2), and has cell-protective properties, especially within the liver. Silybin is the major active ingredient in silymarin and is derived from milk thistle, and has anti-inflammatory activity supporting hepatocytes regeneration, enhances bile flow and production of hepatoprotective bile salts and increases glutathione levels. Unlike SAMe, silybin is not naturally produced by liver cells, and therefore an external nutritional source is required (Table 15.1).

TABLE 15.1 Factors precipitating hepatic encephalopathy (HE).

High-protein meal
GI bleeding or ingestion of blood
Transfusion of stored blood
Constipation
Azotaemia
Metabolic alkalosis
Hypokalaemia
Dietary methionine
Catabolism/hypermetabolism
Sedatives/anaesthetics

CHAPTER 16

Musculoskeletal Disorders

DEVELOPMENTAL ORTHOPAEDIC DISORDERS

Developmental orthopaedic disorders (DOD) involve a diverse group of musculoskeletal disorders that occur in growing animals (most commonly fast-growing large- and giant-breed dogs, and horses) [1]. DODs can be attributed to genetic make-up, nutritional and stress-related aetiologies. This chapter will discuss those aetiologies which are nutritionally induced. The majority of these disorders are made up of canine hip dysplasia (CHD) and dyschondroplasia (DCP) (osteochondrosis dissecans [OCD] is a similar condition but occurs when inflammation is present and a separation of a piece of articular cartilage and the underlying bone within the joint has occurred). Other disorders under the umbrella of DOD include physitis (physeal dysplasia or epiphysitis), angular limb deformities and vertebral abnormalities (Wobbler syndrome). The skeletal system is most susceptible to physical and metabolic insult during the first 12 months of life, due to the heightened metabolic activity [2]. Problems associated with dietary excesses are more likely. Especially in dogs fed a growth food, which is further supplemented with minerals, vitamins and energy sources [3]. Lesions can appear in physeal or articular cartilage as disturbances of endochondral ossification [4].

Nutritional aims:

- Feed a complete and balanced diet, which does not precipitate any predisposition to DODs.
- When DODs do occur, the diet needs to limit any further damage that could be induced through poor or inadequate nutrition.

Clinical Nutrition

Fat

Excessive dietary energy intake may support a growth rate that is too fast for correct skeletal development. Dietary fat is the primary contributor to excess energy intake [2], and therefore, levels should be monitored in large-breed diets, due to fats having twice the calorific density as proteins and carbohydrates. Dietary energy over the animal's requirements will be stored as body fat; therefore, the role of Body Condition Score (BCS) is important to monitor energy intake, alongside the role of growth charts with growth centile lines to help predict and then monitor the growth rates for that individual. Diets aimed at large and giant breeds have a decreased energy density in comparison to small and medium breed puppy diets.

Protein

The proteins used should be of high quality and easily digestible. In dogs, protein excess has not been shown to negatively affect calcium metabolism or skeletal development [1]. A growth diet for dogs should contain >22% protein (Dry Matter Basis (DMB)) of a high biological value [5].

Carbohydrates

The carbohydrate content of the diet does need to be balanced. Levels need to be sufficient to provide adequate calories to the animal, but not excessive to encourage excess weight gain. The type of carbohydrate within the diet is important. In cats and dogs, the carbohydrate content needs to be highly digestible, especially in small breeds of dogs and kittens. In kittens and small breed puppies, high levels of fibre will decrease the digestibility of the diet, and thus they would not be able to consume the calorific quantities required for growth, due to the limited stomach size.

Vitamins and Minerals

The levels of calcium within the diet are vitally important in the development of orthopaedic disorders in large-breed dogs. Equally so is the ratio of calcium to phosphorus present within the diet. Excessive dietary phosphorus consistently produces lesions of dicalcium phosphate (DCP) [5]. An excess of calcium causing hypercalcaemia will result in excess bone deposition, which will interfere with normal bone development.

The roles of vitamin A and D in causing skeletal problems have been well documented. Vitamin A is an essential factor in bone metabolism, especially osteoclastic activity. Deficiencies or excesses in vitamin A can lead to metabolic bone disease, but are fortunately rare due to the use of commercial balanced diets. Vitamin D's metabolites aid in the regulation of calcium metabolism and, therefore, skeletal development. Deficiency of vitamin D (rickets) is rare, again due to the use of commercial diets. Excessive amounts of vitamin D will lead to hypercalcaemia and hyperphosphatemia; clinical signs also include anorexia, polydipsia, polyuria, muscle weakness, generalised soft tissue mineralisation and lameness [1].

Feeding Animals with DODs

The feeding of an animal with or predisposed to DOD must be done on an individual basis, as growth rates and requirements differ greatly. Physical evaluation and BCS should be performed at least every two weeks, with mapping onto a growth curve chart. Care must be given when trying to avoid developmental problems by changing to an adult maintenance diet from a puppy diet, to avoid excess calcium and energy levels. Maintenance foods have a lower energy density than growth diets, so the puppy must consume greater amounts of the diet to reach its energy requirements. Problems can arise if calcium levels in the two diets are similar; the puppy will end up consuming greater amounts of calcium than if fed the growth diet.

Guidance should be given to owners that calcium supplements should not be given to growing puppies unless prescribed by a veterinary surgeon. Owners should be made aware of the risk of DOD, and that commercial growth diets contain all the required calcium needed.

If a DOD has occurred, then a review of the animal's diet and BCS is required. Nutrition can be used to aid in the prevention of DOD, but its role once it has been acquired is limited. It should always be remembered that food manufacturers' recommendations are just that; reassessment of the animal over regular periods is the best method in obtaining a feeding plan and the method by which the animal is being fed, with completion of growth curve charts (Figure 16.1 and Table 16.1).

OSTEOARTHRITIS

Osteoarthritis (OA) can be an exceptionally painful and crippling disease. OA or degenerative joint disease (DJD) is a chronic progressive disease characterised by pathological changes in the movable joints. Dietary manipulation can aid in the management of arthritis and help improve the animal's mobility. Arthritis can be divided into two classifications:

1. Degenerative types of arthritis, in which the degradation of the articular cartilage is a prominent feature.
2. Inflammatory arthropathies, where synovitis is the main pathological feature.

OA is the most common form of arthritis experienced in both animals and humans. Management of OA includes weight (obesity) control, appropriate exercise management, and anti-inflammatory medications. OA is characterised by degeneration of the articular cartilage and proliferation of new bone.

With the multiplicity of drugs and alternative treatments utilised for chronic pain, management of these patients can be difficult and complex. It's important to emphasise to the owners of these pets that multiple trials may be required to find the right combination of analgesics, supplements and diets, and that not all patients can be effectively managed.

Obesity is a major risk factor and contributor to OA. Weight loss (at all stages) must be initiated as soon as possible. Exercising and consequently weight loss can be difficult due to restrictions in mobility. When deciding on a diet for an animal with OA, it needs to meet the requirements for the animal's life stage and body condition score.

It has been reported that 90% of cats and dogs over the age of 12 years old have shown to have changes in their bones, suggesting OA when radiographed.

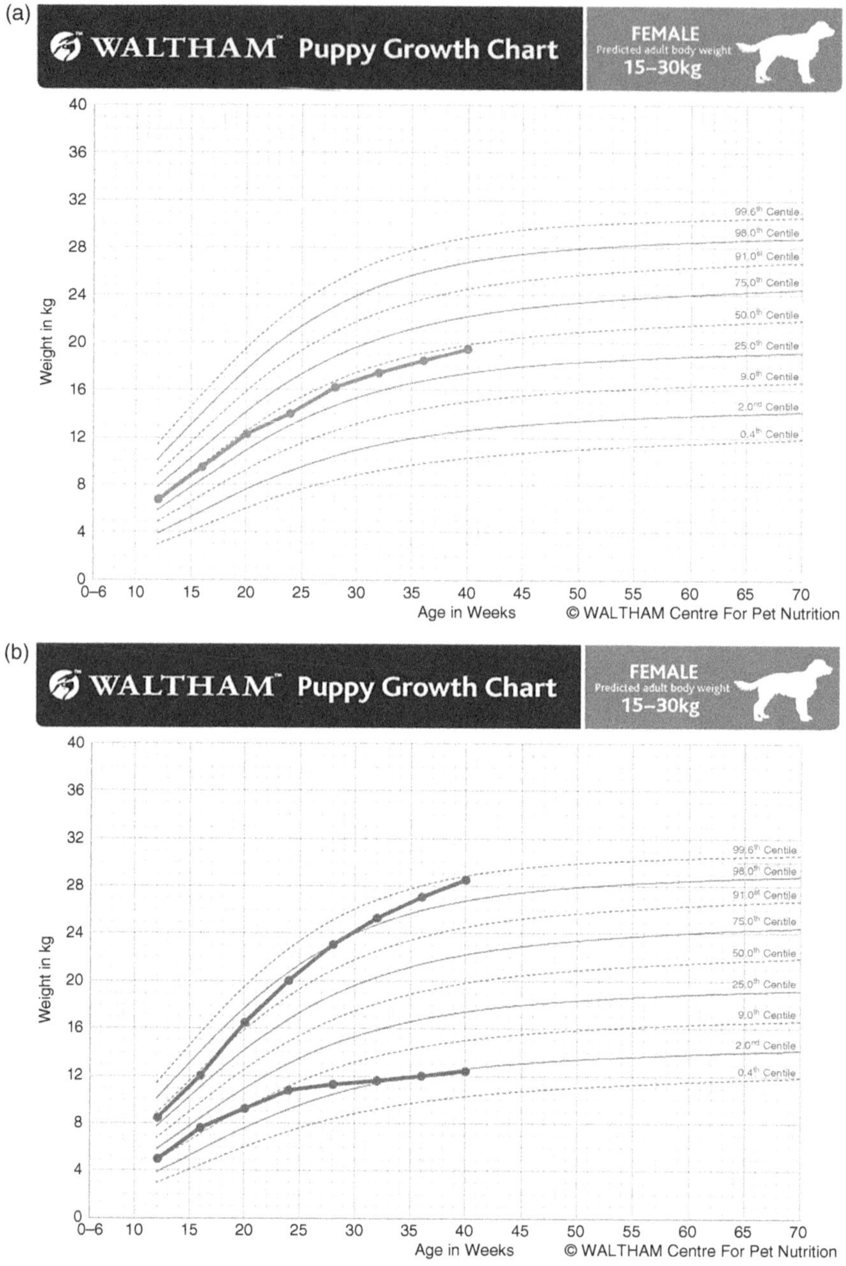

FIGURE 16.1 (a) Growth chart showing an ideal growth curve, staying within the percentile lines. (b) Growth chart showing growth rates that have either grown too quickly or too slowly, crossing two percentile lincs. With permission of Mars or Affiliates.

TABLE 16.1 Key points for nutrition for animals with DOD.

Ensure a correct calcium-phosphorus ratio.
Feed a controlled energy level, suitable for the individual.
Regularly assess weight and BCS.
Use of a growth chart is advisable in the monitoring of growth rates.

Nutraceuticals

These are nutrients that are administered at a high enough level to have positive effects in the body. The main nutraceuticals used for arthritis are the omega-3 EFA, eicosapentaenoic acid (EPA) and docosahexaenoic acid (DHA). The use of chondroprotectants and other nutraceuticals has become commonplace for cats and dogs suffering from OA. Chondroprotective agents are reported to have three primary effects:

1. Anabolic, by supporting or enhancing the metabolism of chondrocytes and synoviocytes.
2. Catabolic, inhibits degradative enzymes within the synovial fluid and cartilage matrix.
3. Antithrombolic, inhibits the formation of thrombi in small blood vessels supplying the joint [1].

Nutraceuticals are a branch of chondroprotective agents and are defined as a non-drug substance that is produced in a purified or extracted form and administered orally to provide compounds required for normal body structure and function, with the intent of improving health and well-being. Different types of nutraceuticals used in the management of OA are described below.

Fatty Acids

OA is a common radiographic finding in older cats, with a prevalence of up to 90% in appendicular joints [6]. A randomised, controlled, double-blinded prospective clinical study examined a diet high in fish oil, green-lipped mussel extract and glucosamine/chondroitin in client-owned osteoarthritic cats. The authors found that osteoarthritic cats receiving the diet, as compared with a control group, were more active as measured objectively with a collar-mounted accelerometer over a nine-week period [7]. Although this is not direct evidence of improvement, it was theorised that increased activity reflected decreased pain associated with OA.

EPA is the most effective *n*-3 polyunsaturated fatty acid (PUFA) for preventing cartilage catabolism in in vitro models. This data would suggest that supplementation of food with EPA would prove to be beneficial in slowing the rate of cartilage degradation in canine DJD. EPA blocks the genes that produce the cartilage-degrading enzymes aggrecanase and matrix metalloproteinases (MMPs). These enzymes cause progression of the disease, even continuing after the absence of inflammation. For example, if the animal is medicated with non-steroidal anti-inflammatory drugs (NSAIDs). NSAIDs stop inflammation that is caused by chondrocyte damage, but it does not stop degradation. The symptoms of OA are being controlled, but as the damage continues, gradual increases in medication will be required. EPA is the only omega-3 (*n*-3) fatty acid that is taken up by chondrocytes and remains active within the joint. EPA also helps soothe the inflammation associated with OA. Use of diets enriched with EPA has shown that the dose of NSAIDs required to control clinical signs in dogs with OA could be reduced [1].

The ratio of fatty acids is of great importance. High levels of omega-3 and a low ratio of omega-6 are required.

Glucosamine

Glucosamine supplements are the most commonly used within the OA market, and glucosamine hydrochloride or glucosamine sulphate are the most commonly found. Of the two, glucosamine hydrochloride will yield more glucosamine per unit weight than the sulphate form to the animal. This should be clearly explained to the owner who may wish to purchase non-veterinary products, which appear cheaper. Glucosamine is a precursor to glycosaminoglycans (GAGs), which are present in the extracellular matrix of articular cartilage. When damage occurs to chondrocytes, there is a decreased ability to synthesise glucosamine; supplementing the diet stimulates the production of proteoglycans and collagen by these cells.

In traumatic DJD, the natural balance between synthesis and degradation of cartilage shifts towards increasing degradation, resulting in loss of mucopolysaccharides. Commercially used products are chemically similar to the mucopolysaccharides of the articular cartilage, and it is concentrated in the cartilaginous tissue.

Chondroitin sulphate (CS) is another GAG present within the extracellular matrix of the articular cartilage. CS has been shown to stimulate the production of proteoglycans and collagen, like glucosamine, but can also inhibit histamine-mediated inflammation, decrease interleukin-1 production and inhibit metalloproteinases.

Boswellia serrata is a branching tree native to the hilly regions of India. It produces an aromatic resin that is used for medicinal purposes. Boswellia resin administered for six weeks in dogs helped to reduce lameness (when moving or after a long rest), local pain and stiff gait [4]. The anti-inflammatory effects of Boswellia and boswellic acids have been linked to the ability to inhibit the synthesis of leukotrienes [8], the chemical mediators of the inflammatory process in various inflammatory diseases, including arthritis [9].

UC-II collagen for canines is an undenatured type II collagen, a key structural component of healthy cartilage, that is clinically proven to improve joint health in dogs. It works by supporting joint function and cartilage preservation, which is particularly beneficial for older dogs or those with existing joint issues. UC-II is derived from chicken sternum cartilage using a patented process that maintains its natural 3D structure. An oral intake of small amounts of glycosylated UC-II® presents active epitopes, with the correct three-dimensional structures, to the Peyer's patches; this process triggers the signalling required for the development of immune tolerance [5]. The UC-II® has demonstrated the ability to induce this tolerance, effectively reducing joint pain and swelling in rheumatoid arthritis subjects [5, 10]. It is believed to engage the immune system and the joint cartilage metabolism: UC-II® can alleviate T-cell response and activate T-regulatory cells via its oral tolerance mechanism, which eventually may reduce cartilage damage.

Egg shell membrane (ESM), found between the calcified shell and the albumin in chicken eggs, is primarily composed of fibrous proteins such as collagen type I [11], which form the mesh-like structure of the bilayer material. However, ESMs have also been shown to contain other bioactive components, namely glycosaminoglycans (i.e. dermatan sulphate [6], CS [7], hyaluronic acid [12], etc.). ESM is known to reduce the expression of various proinflammatory cytokines both in vitro [13] and in vivo [13], including the key mediators of inflammation, interleukin-1 beta and tumour necrosis factor-alpha.

Postoperative Uses

All surgery performed on any joint will induce some level of OA. The use of chondroprotectants has been encouraged in the postoperative period and during the physical rehabilitation period to accelerate and enhance recovery. Periods of immobilisation should be discouraged, as a reduction in synovial fluid production and proteoglycan depletion occurs due to the reduction in loading on the joint. The use of chondroprotectants aids in pain relief, so that the animal is more likely to perform physiotherapy exercises, it reduces the degradative and inflammatory enzymes which help protect the cartilage and stimulates the synovial fluid, proteoglycan and collagen production to promote cartilage matrix repair.

REFERENCES

1. Beale, B.S. (2004). Use of nutraceuticals and chondroprotectants in osteoarthritic dogs and cats. *Vet. Clin. North Am. Small Anim. Pract.* 34 (1): 271–290.
2. May, S.A. (1996). Current research relevant to equine joint disease: animal models and other experimental systems in the investigation of equine arthritis. In: *Joint Disease in the Horse* (ed. C.W. McIlwraith and G. Trotter). Philadelphia: Saunders.
3. McIlwraith, C.W. and Vachon, A. (1998). Review of pathogenesis and treatment of degenerative joint disease. *Eq. Vet. J. Suppl.* 6: 3–11.
4. Comblain, F., Serisier, S., Barthelemy, N. et al. (2015). Review of dietary supplements for the management of osteoarthritis in dogs in studies from 2004 to 2014. *J. Vet. Pharmacol. Ther.* 39: 1–15.
5. Bagchi, D., Misner, B., Bagchi, M. et al. (2002). Effects of orally administered undenatured type-II collagen against arthritic inflammatory diseases: a mechanistic exploration. *Int. J. Clin. Pharmacol. Res.* 22 (3–4): 101–110.
6. Baker, J.R. and Balch, D.A. (1962). A study of the organic material of hen's-egg shell. *Biochem. J.* 82: 352–361.
7. Long, F.D., Adams, R.G., and DeVore, D.P. (2005). Inventors. Preparation of hyaluronic acid from eggshell membrane. 69465512005920. `https://pubchem.ncbi.nlm.nih.gov/patent/US-6946551-B2#section=Filing-Date`
8. Reichling, J., Schmokel, H., Fitzi, J. et al. (2004). Dietary support with Boswellia resin in canine inflammatory joint and spinal disease. *Schweiz. Arch. Tierheilkd.* 146: 71–79.
9. Kimmatkar, N., Thawani, V., Hingorani, L., and Khiyani, R. (2003). Efficacy and tolerability of *Boswellia serrata* extract in treatment of osteoarthritis of knee – a randomized double-blind placebo controlled trial. *Phytomedicine* 10: 3–7.
10. Stabile, M., Samarelli, R., Trerotoli, P. et al. (2019). Evaluation of the effects of undenatured type-II collagen (UC-II) as compared to robenacoxib on the mobility impairment induced by osteoarthritis in dogs. *Vet. Sci.* 6 (3): 72.

11. Wong, M., Hendrix, M.J.C., von der Mark, K. et al. (1984). Collagen in the egg shell membranes of the hen. *Dev. Biol.* 104 (1): 28–36.
12. Benson, K.F., Ruff, K.J., and Jensen, G.S. (2012). Effects of natural eggshell membrane (NEM) on cytokine production in cultures of peripheral blood mononuclear cells: increased suppression of tumor necrosis factor-α levels after in vitro digestion. *J. Med. Food* 15 (4): 360–368.
13. Ruff, K.J. and DeVore, D.P. (2014). Reduction of pro-inflammatory cytokines in rats following 7-day oral supplementation with a proprietary eggshell membrane-derived product. *Mod. Res. Inflamm.* 3 (1): 31003.

CHAPTER 17

Obesity

Obesity is a complex, chronic medical condition that needs to be managed throughout the life of the individual patient. All elements of a weight-management plan should be discussed with the client: nutrition, behaviour and exercise. Aims of clinical nutrition include:

- Supply adequate nutrients within a reduced-calorie diet.
- Promote smooth weight loss, whilst maintaining a lean body mass as much as possible.
- Increase conversion of stored fat to energy.

PREVENTION OF OBESITY

Prevention is better than cure, and the ideal place to start is in puppy and kitten nurse clinics, first vaccinations and during socialisation and training groups. It has been clearly demonstrated that animals that remain at or marginally below their ideal weight throughout their growth phase are less likely to become obese in later life (Figure 17.1) [1].

The graph tracks 48 Labrador Retrievers over 14 years, split into two groups:

- Control Dogs (Gold Line): These dogs were allowed to eat more (often 'free-choice' as puppies). They had higher body fat and reached a median life span of 11.2 years.
- Lean-fed Dogs (Dark Green Line): These dogs were fed 25% less than their siblings. They maintained an 'ideal' lean body condition and lived to a median age of 13.0 years.

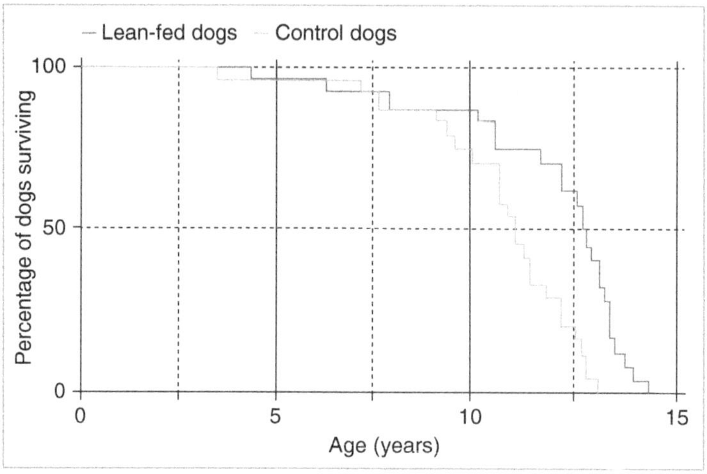

FIGURE 17.1 Purina Life Span Study. Adapted from [1].

The key findings from this study highlighted a lifespan extension: The lean-fed dogs lived a median of 1.8 years (15%) longer than the control group. There was also an increase in health span. Beyond just living longer, the lean-fed dogs showed a delayed onset of chronic diseases. For example, clinical signs of osteoarthritis were delayed by an average of three years. Ageing Signs: Lean-fed dogs exhibited fewer visible signs of ageing, such as greying muzzles and impaired gaits, at a much later age.

Following up on puppies/kittens post-neutering is vital; this also includes when chemical castration methods have been utilised. With a decrease in metabolism and a change in diet, many animals do tend to increase their weight and body condition score (BCS) at this stage in life and subsequently battle with it into adulthood. The VN is the ideal person to discuss postoperative changes in diet and feeding amounts. Why not encourage all animals to see a VN at intervals throughout the growth phase to monitor weight and BCS and to discuss diet/feeding? Many owners find the timings for transitioning to junior or adult and whether to use a neutered diet quite confusing.

Risk Factors

Where we know that there are higher risk factors for obesity (age, breed, neuter status and concurrent disease), discussion with owners surrounding caloric intake should occur. Breed in dogs does significantly affect the occurrence ratio (OR) of obesity (Box 17.1). In this table, a Cavalier King Charles Spaniel has an OR of 5.174; this means that they are 5.174 times more likely to be overweight or obese than the control group, which in this case was dogs registered onto the practices' computer system as a crossbreed dog.

The same study also identified that gender in dogs is a risk factor. Females are more likely than males to be overweight/obese (OR 1.49; $p < 0.001$). Age was also a risk factor. Risk increases with age in dogs (OR 1.07; $p < 0.001$). This is the opposite for cats, where over the age of 11 years, cats will start to decline in weight due to a reduction in nutrient assimilation.

Box 17.1 Occurrence ratios of various breeds: their likelihood of becoming obese

Border Terrier (OR 3.122, $p < 0.001$)
Cairn Terrier (OR 3.217, $p < 0.01$)
CKCS (OR 5.174, $p < 0.001$)
Chihuahua (OR 3.945, $p < 0.01$)
Cocker Spaniel (OR 2.249, $p < 0.001$)
Dachshund (OR 4.448, $p < 0.001$)
German/Belgian Shepherd (OR 0.188, $p < 0.001$)
Pointer/Vizala/Weimaraner (OR 0.312, $p = 0.005$)
Labrador (OR 0.647, $p < 0.01$)
Golden Retriever (OR 0.529, $p < 0.01$)
Setters (OR 0.362, $p < 0.05$)
Rottweiler (OR 0.218, $p < 0.001$)

Obesity is the most prevalent form of malnutrition in pets presented to veterinary practices. Obesity is defined as when body fat exceeds 15–20% of body weight [1]. Excessive weight is an associated cause or exacerbating factor for specific orthopaedic, endocrine, cardiovascular and neoplastic diseases [2]. Obesity will also make the animal less tolerant or resilient to metabolic stress. The weight and volume of fat in the abdomen of an obese animal can exert enough pressure on the bladder to induce leakage of urine but also to reduce the diameter of the urethra and cause reduced flow of urine. The animal ultimately needs to change from a positive energy balance to a negative energy balance in order to lose and then maintain an ideal body weight.

CLINICAL NUTRITION

Satiation is related to the rate of food consumption (animals can overeat before realising that they are satiated), food constituents (protein is more satiating than carbohydrates) and the animal's sense of fullness. These three factors should be used in the construction of a dietary plan for obesity control. Nutritional management only comprises part of a weight loss management programme; the animal's metabolism (clinical history), exercise levels and lifestyle also need to be considered.

Protein

Diets with high-protein levels can be classed as low-energy diets, in comparison to those that are high in carbohydrates (Table 17.1). These diets can be advantageous, as they conserve lean body mass whilst being efficient in inducing weight loss in cats.

TABLE 17.1 Calorific value of nutrients.

	1 g carbohydrate	1 g protein	1 g fat
GE	4.2 kcal	5.4 kcal	9.4 kcal
GE → DE			
	3.7 kcal 88%	4.8 kcal 89%	8.5 kcal 90%
DE → ME			
	3.5 kcal 83%	3.5 kcal 65%	8.5 kcal 90%
ME → NE			
True energy value % of GE	3.2 kcal 76%	2.2 kcal 41%	8.2 kcal 87%

Values stated as kcal per gram are usually of metabolised energy and not the net energy gained by the diet. By using the net energy fraction, calorie differences are greater. This highlights the advantages of using a high-protein diet in cats [3].

Protein levels are also an important element of weight loss diets, as the preservation of lean muscle mass is important. Preserving lean muscle mass during weight loss in pets is best achieved through a high-protein, restricted-calorie diet combined with gradual, controlled weight loss (approx. 1–2% body weight/week). Increasing protein intake helps protect muscle tissue, prevents metabolic rate decline and ensures fat loss. Feeding high-protein, low-fat diets (30–40% protein on a metabolisable energy basis) has been shown to result in significantly more fat loss and less muscle loss in dogs and cats. Monitoring muscle condition score (MCS) during the weight loss period is advocated.

Carbohydrates

The role of carbohydrates in an obesity diet can be vital. The method in which obesity diets work can be altering the levels of non-fermentable fibres. The role of the fibre is to achieve the sensation of satiety in the animal whilst the animal receives a reduced proportion of calories within its diet. In some high-fibre obesity diets, this can mean that only 60–70% of the animal's daily calorific requirement is obtained from the diet. The subsequent 30–40% is obtained from the utilisation of the animal's bodily fat reserves. High-fibre diets, in cats, may affect object play and therefore reduce calorie expenditure. Exercise regimes as part of a calorie-controlled diet are important to help retain lean body mass.

Prebiotic fibres play a crucial role in canine appetite management by promoting satiety, increasing faecal bulk, and stimulating the release of gut hormones that signal fullness, such as PYY and GLP-1. These nondigestible carbohydrates, including fructooligosaccharides (FOS), galactooligosaccharides (GOS) and soluble corn fibre (SCF), are fermented in the colon to produce short-chain fatty acids (SCFAs), which help regulate intestinal motility and reduce hunger.

This high level of fibre can have its disadvantages, which should be clearly explained to the owner if the weight loss plan is to be successful. These disadvantages include the increase in faecal output and possibly flatulence.

Fats

The fat level in an obesity diet doesn't necessarily need to be restricted in order to control calorific intake. The diet should, however, contain the necessary levels of the EFA. Some obesity diets aid in weight loss by only providing the animal with ~60–70% of their daily energy requirements. The required energy shortfall is met by the utilisation of the animal's bodily fat stores.

Vitamins and Minerals

The oxidative cell damage that is caused by free radicals is higher in obese animals than in those that are lean. It is therefore recommended that the diet be supplemented with higher levels of antioxidants. If comparing diets on a calorific value, the vitamin and mineral levels in these diets will seem higher. This is due to the low-calorie nature of the diet. When comparing nutrient levels in these diets, it is advisable to use other quantitative values. The typical vitamin and mineral values should be sufficient for the life stage of that particular individual.

L-Carnitine

L-Carnitine (β-hydroxy-γ-trimethylaminobutyric acid) is a small water-soluble vitamin-like molecule [4]. L-Carnitine is concentrated in mammalian cardiac and skeletal muscle by an active membrane transport mechanism. L-Carnitine has been shown to increase body fat loss and prevent loss of muscle mass [5]. L-Carnitine can also protect cats from hepatic lipid accumulation during calorie restriction [6]. Most veterinary clinical obesity diets do contain supplemented levels of L-carnitine.

Nutrigenomics in Obesity

- Diet affects genes: Obese dogs fed a high-fibre, low-fat therapeutic veterinary food showed a down-regulation (turning off) of genes associated with inflammation and obesity and an upregulation of genes that promote a lean profile.
- Nutrients affecting metabolic pathways: In canine obesity, specialised nutrients in therapeutic foods have been shown to modulate the expression of genes involved in fat storage and insulin sensitivity, such as Peroxisome Proliferator-Activated Receptor Alpha (*PPARA*) and Lipoprotein Lipase (*LPL*).
- Genotype affects response: A study showed that cats with different genetic markers might respond differently to high-fat diets, with some individuals having a genetic predisposition to higher fat accumulation, requiring specific weight-loss strategies.

- Metabolic gene expression: In weight-loss studies, it was observed that in obese dogs, the expression of genes responsible for inflammation and fat accumulation was reduced after dietary intervention, shifting their metabolism toward a leaner phenotype (physical appearance).

There are veterinary diets that utilise ingredients that help in the upregulation of genes associated with metabolism and thus aid weight loss and the preservation of lean muscle mass.

Feeding an Obesity Diet

Weight reduction programmes initiated within the veterinary practice do tend to be more successful, mainly due to close monitoring and the support offered. Programmes include three important stages. A feeding plan, based on the amount of excess fat to lose and what is currently being fed; an exercise plan, based on mobility allowances and the owner's lifestyle and job commitments; and a recheck plan. Reduced-calorie intake alone will not substantially reduce weight. For the weight reduction to be a success, all three stages of the programme must be completed. Stage 3, the recheck plan, will depend on the case history, the success of weight loss and the practice policy. In many cases, a recheck every two weeks is normal.

In order to correctly design a feeding plan, the ideal body weight of the animal needs to be obtained. An ideal or optimal body weight should be calculated by examining the animal. Using BCS is the preferred way to assess the animal as it takes into account the animal's frame size independent of its weight. The animal's coat can also prove to be quite deceptive in obscuring an underweight or overweight animal. Dogs and cats that have an optimal BCS have normal body contours; the bony prominences can be palpated readily under the skin surfaces. Looking back over the animal's previous weight history can aid in identifying the ideal body weight. If the animal had an ideal BCS earlier in its life, you can use this, or if the owner states that at one year of age the animal was at its ideal body weight, this can be used. Once an ideal body weight has been calculated, the amount of weight to be lost is now known. Some therapeutic or prescription diets require the animal to be fed a set amount depending on the ideal body weight and adjusted thereafter from this quantity in 10% increments. Evaluating the animal's diet and removing all titbits and snacks will aid in an initial loss of weight. This strategy will have limited weight loss in most animals. Reduction in quantities of a maintenance diet can lead to deficiencies in important nutrients and should be avoided.

All weight loss diets have their advantages and disadvantages, and any disadvantages of using high-fibre diets should be explained to the owners. Increases in defecation and faecal output, if not explained to the owner, can cause the owner to cease feeding the diet. Encouraging the owner to feed the last daily diet earlier and giving the animal more access to either the litter tray or the ability to go outside will eliminate any problems. The correct ratio is to feed 60% of the maintenance rate for the animal's body weight. Fat will then be utilised to provide the shortfall supply.

Once the ideal weight has been achieved, maintaining this optimal weight can be difficult, and even more frequent weight checkups may be required. Owner encouragement is still recommended to keep up established exercise regimes and positive feeding habits, as lost weight can easily be regained. Dogs and cats do experience a 'rebound' effect post-weight loss if fed an uncontrolled diet [7]. Selection of a new diet once the optimal weight has been achieved can be difficult and can vary from animal to animal. Some will maintain the optimal weight well on a light life-stage diet, combined with an exercise programme. Others will require a modified amount of the obesity diet or a transitional therapeutic weight control diet [8].

The length of time required to reach optimal weight does depend on the individual patient. It can be calculated by:

$$\frac{\text{Initial bwt (g)} - \text{Target bwt (g)}}{\text{Weekly weight loss (g)}} = \text{Time to reach target bwt (weeks).}$$

The weekly weight loss can differ from week to week, especially in cats whose activity levels can vary greatly, especially dependent on the weather. In multi-cat households, there is often one fat cat and one or more lean cats. Play and activity feeding should be emphasised. The use of tunnels or small holes for feeding access, which the fat cat can't get through, can be utilised for the leaner cats.

BEHAVIOUR AND ITS ROLE IN OBESITY

Behaviour plays an important role in obesity and should be addressed with the owner. This involves behavioural interactions between other animals in the household and between the owner and the animal. Cats can easily become obese due to overeating in a multi-cat household. In these situations, cats need to have their own safe feeding station. Each feeding station needs to be separate from the litter tray and from their own water bowl. There needs to be a greater number of water bowls and feeding bowls than the number of cats in the household, all of these in different positions. In the majority of cases, the obese cat in the multi-cat household is the cat that is the most nervous one. Cat behaviour is very difficult for owners to interrupt, and many do not perceive that there is a tension in the air between their own cats. Cats can be known to binge eat when other cats are not present near the feeding bowl. Owners can interrupt this as the obese cat does not eat much as it only goes to the bowl very infrequently, normally when the owners are not there, and eats very fast. This can result in the overall amount of calories being taken on board being higher than normal. In these cases, it can be useful to have a 'safe room' in the house for the nervous cat. The cat can be fed separately away from the other cats and eat at its own pace. This feeding regime can also be utilised for cats suffering from FLUTD, as the reduction in stress can help in the prevention of recurrence.

Cats have adapted to eat little and often, and changing the cat to a meal-based feeding can be difficult. Owners should be encouraged to weigh out the daily rations of food on weighing scales. This allocated amount of diet can then be used throughout the day to feed the cat little and often. Encouraging the cat to exercise is always recommended; throwing single kibbles for the cat to eat will encourage movement. The use of light beams is also beneficial, but after chasing the light around, the light should always end on a toy that the cat can pouch on and attach. This satisfies the cat's hunting behaviour and will prevent the cat from becoming frustrated in the play behaviour.

Discuss with the owner that the cat's behaviour is not normal – lying around the house all day and night is not normal for a cat.

The main behavioural element regarding obesity in dogs is the giving and receiving of treats. Weight loss is not just about nutrition and exercise regimes. It is mainly about human psychology; any veterinary nurse that runs clinics will tell you this. Feeding = love, and it is an opportunity to interact and exchange affection and touch, it is deemed a fun activity. We all know that dieting is not fun, and owners perceive this in their pets; hungry means unhappy, which equates to losing love. If dieting were easy, we would all be slim, but it is not, it is difficult. Dieting requires changing habits, which can be uncomfortable and difficult. Internally, the owner requires motivation, but externally, support is also required, the ideal role for the veterinary nurse.

PHARMACEUTICALS

The use of pharmaceuticals can also affect canine behaviour. Whilst not entirely understood, the proposed mechanisms of microsomal triglyceride transfer protein (MTP) inhibitors in weight loss include both inhibition of dietary lipid absorption across the intestine and stimulation of gut hormones that signal satiety (e.g. GLP-1 and PYY). The use of pharmaceuticals can aid those owners who have difficulty coping with begging behaviour from their dogs. Potential problems can arise when owners feel that their pets no longer love them, as the dog is not greeting them at the door when they come home from work. Owners mistake this behaviour as a greeting rather than the dog looking for a food source. When a food-oriented dog has the drive for food removed, it will alter its behaviour greatly. Owners should be informed of these possible changes. Rewards for the dog need to be altered from food to another form of reward. Interactions from the owner have tended to be the handing over of a treat, and then the dog returns to whatever it was doing beforehand. Encouraging the owner to play with the dog, grooming the dog, and taking the dog out for a walk are all methods of different interactions that the owner can undertake. Ongoing weight management is required as discontinuation of the drugs results in the return of appetite and weight gain if food intake is not controlled.

During the period of time that the dog is receiving the pharmaceuticals, any undesired behaviours associated with food need to be addressed, both from the dog's point of view and the owner's behaviour.

Tips for Weight Loss

It can be useful to have a printed list of top tips to give to the owner when starting out on the weight loss programme. Most reiterate what would have already been covered during the process of the obesity clinic but also aid in the compliance of the owner to attend clinics.

- Have regular weight checks with a pet slimmer's clinic/nurse. Regular contact with the pet slimmer's nurse can dramatically help with your pet's weight loss. Feeding quantities may need adjusting in order to find the correct amount for your pet.

- Weigh out the daily food allowance in the morning and place it in a container. Use this food for the allocated meals; this way, it is less likely to overfeed. You can take out a few kibbles to use as treats throughout the day.
- Increase exercise levels gently; it is important for the pet slimmer's nurse to help design an exercise programme. Little and often can prove to be more beneficial for weight loss. Cats can exercise by use of toys, light torches, etc., and always ensure that this play activity ends on an object. This will satisfy the cat's hunting activities, and they won't get frustrated.
- Placing the food in different areas or hiding kibbles around the house/room can encourage cats to exercise more. Use of a food ball is ideal in these situations.
- If you have more than one cat, it is important to feed them separately and to observe them when they are eating.
- It can be wise to inform your neighbours that your pet is going on a weight loss programme and not to feed it.
- For a weight loss programme to be successful, everyone involved in caring for the pet, or that may feed the pet, needs to be involved and 'on board'.
- It is important that no 'extras' are added to your pet's daily allocated allowance. This also includes all forms of milk, broths and soups.

REFERENCES

1. Kealy, R. D., Lawler, D. F., Ballam, J. M., Mantz, S. L., Biery, D. N., Greeley, E. H., Lust, G., Segre, M., Smith, G. K., & Stowe, H. D. (2002). Effects of diet restriction on life span and age-related changes in dogs. *J. Am. Vet. Med. Assoc.*, 220 (9): 1315–1320. https://doi.org/10.2460/javma.2002.220.1315
2. Debraekaleer, J. (2004). Obesity in cats and dogs. *Veterinary Times* (22nd March), p. 14.
3. Biourge, V. (2001). *Obesity, a Major Risk Factor for Diabetes in Cats. Royal Canin's Guide to Feline Obesity*, 10–13. Royal Canin Publications.
4. Martin, L. (2001). *The Principle of High-Protein Diets and Net Energy. Royal Canin's Guide to Feline Obesity*, 6–9. Royal Canin Publications.
5. Pion, P.D. (2004). Traditional and non-traditional effective and noneffective therapies for cardiac disease in dogs and cats. *Vet. Clin. Small Animal* 34: 187–216.
6. Armstrong, P.J., Hardie, E.M. and Cullen, J.M. (1992). L-Carnitine reduces hepatic fat accumulation during rapid weight reduction in cats. *Proceedings of the 10th Veterinary Medical Forum*, 810.
7. Gross, K.L., Wedekind, K.J. and Kirk, C.A. (1998). Effect of dietary carnitine or chromium on weight loss and body composition of obese dogs. *Proceedings of the American Society of Animal Science.*
8. LaFlamme DP and Kuhlman G. The effect of weight loss on subsequent weight maintenance in dogs. *J. Vet. Intern. Med.* 1993; 7 (134): 1019–1028. doi: https://doi.org/10.1016/0271-5317(95)00063-O.

CHAPTER 18

Chronic Renal Disease

INTRODUCTION

The nutrition of those with renal disease can be complex and very dependent on the patients (cats or dogs). A nutritional assessment should be performed on all patients at every appropriate point of contact, comprising weight, body condition score (BCS), muscle condition score (MCS) and nutrition history (what, where and how they eat, including behavioural aspects, as these are especially important in patients). Blood and urine parameters are required to stage the renal disease and to give the correct nutritional advice.

Energy Requirements

The proposed nutritional requirements for senior cats and dogs were traditionally fewer calories (as they are more inactive), lower protein levels, softer kibbles and reduced sodium and phosphorus in the diet. The ageing factors of senior cats have led to the conclusion that the energy requirements in cats alter and can increase once geriatric stages are reached [1]. This does differ from dogs that don't have a reduction in their ability to digest and therefore utilise the diet. Different stages of senior life will require different energy requirements, alongside different disease processes, and a possible reduction in activity if osteoarthritis is present will also influence energy requirements. Recommendations are made that the nutritional assessment be undertaken to assess these energy requirements. Renal diets, due to the reduction in protein levels, will have a percentage shift in carbohydrate and fat quantities. Care needs to be taken in dogs that have a predisposition, previous clinical history, or even breed risk for pancreatitis with those diets that have a relative increase in fat levels.

Protein Requirements

A reduction in protein quantities within the diet could be beneficial if renal damage has occurred [2], though this is dependent on the International Renal Interest Society (IRIS) staging of the chronic kidney disease (CKD). The quality (the biological value [BV]) of the protein should be increased as skeletal muscle mass reduces, which also reduces any protein or amino acid reserves. Protein restriction in feline and canine senior and renal diets should be avoided until IRIS stages 2–4, due to the potential decrease in lean muscle mass. Cats are especially sensitive to decreases in protein levels within the diet. This is due to the inability to downregulate protein metabolism pathways. Reduced fat digestibility is also experienced in geriatric cats [3]. In healthy adult cats, protein digestibility is typically 85–90%. In geriatric cats, this digestibility can be reduced to less than 77%. Diets, which have a severely restricted protein level or proteins of low quality/BV, can predispose cats over 12 years to negative nitrogen balance and loss of lean body mass [3]. All animals with renal impairment need close monitoring for this. MCS is vital but can be difficult as it is based on palpation. Maintaining the balance between the quantity and quality of the proteins and the potential waste products is required.

The restriction of phosphorus in the diet does play a significant role in the prevention of renal impairment [4]. The level of restriction does depend on the IRIS staging (see Table 18.1).

A decrease in kidney function can also lead to an increased loss of the water-soluble vitamins due to the kidneys' decreased ability to concentrate the urine. This can also lead to a reduction in the hydration levels of the animal. Senior animals have a reduced sensitivity to thirst, and thus there is a greater risk of dehydration in these animals.

TABLE 18.1 IRIS staging, phosphate levels and dietary recommendations.

IRIS staging	IRIS stage 1 UPCR < 0.4 (cats) and <0.5 (dogs) Serum phosphate <1.5 mmol/l	IRIS stage 1 And/or proteinuria of renal origin with UPCR >0.4 (cats) and >0.5 (dogs); and/or serum phosphorus >1.5 mmol/l	IRIS stages 2–4 And/or proteinuria of renal origin with UPCR >0.4 (cats and dogs); and/or serum phosphorus >1.5 mmol/l
Aim for a serum phosphate target of mmol/l	0.81–1.45	0.81–1.61	0.81–1.94
Nutritional management recommendations	**Senior diets** Look for high EPA-DHA content and low phosphate.	**Early renal diets** Look for protein levels similar to senior diets with good/high digestibility.	**Advanced renal diets** Phosphate binders may be required where the animal isn't consuming a low-phosphate diet or the renal disease is advanced and not able to be controlled on the renal diet alone.

DHA, docosahexaenoic acid; EPA, eicosapentaenoic acid; and UPCR, Urine protein creatinine ratio.

Water

Increasing water consumption can be achieved in several different ways. Feeding a moist diet rather than a dry diet and increasing the availability of water. Increasing the number of bowls (including types) around the house and allowing water to stand for some time before being offered to some animals can be beneficial. This allows the chlorine in the water to evaporate off, which some animals do prefer. Use of water fountains can also help to increase water intake. Ideally, phosphate-free hydration broths that can aid in increasing calorific intake alongside hydration without an increase in phosphate. As part of the nursing clinic, it is important to discuss with the client how to monitor hydration levels. Demonstrating monitoring of clinical signs can help the client in the care of their pet. This can include testing for skin tenting, tacky mucus membranes and the colour of membranes. If pet owners know what is normal, when the animal becomes unwell or the renal disease progresses, they can flag this to the practice more quickly. Ultimately, increasing the welfare of the animal.

As the animal ages, smell is the first sense to decline. As the animal's sense of smell deteriorates, the animal may eat less. The aroma of the diet is particularly important in diets aimed at senior animals to encourage consumption. Wet diets do smell more than dry, though it should be remembered that cat's dietary preference is also based on the texture of the diet [5].

Diets supplemented with antioxidants, prebiotics and fatty acids had significantly higher average serum vitamin E levels and significantly better-maintained body weight and lean body mass, skin thickness and haematocrit values in comparison to cats on the control diet, as well as a more beneficial faecal microbiota balance. Overall quality of life did appear better but wasn't measured [6].

FIBRE AND THE MICROBIOME

Some manufacturers of renal diets don't emphasise the importance of dietary fibre for this clinical condition. The animal itself cannot digest soluble/fermentable fibre in the diet, but the microbes within the intestine can. Soluble fibre is fermented into short-chain fatty acids (SCFAs) or volatile fatty acids (VFAs). These products are an important energy source for the intestinal cells and can increase blood flow to the intestine.

Nitrogenous waste products in the blood are presented to the intestinal lumen, where urease, an enzyme produced by intestinal bacteria, hydrolyses the urea into ammonia and carbon dioxide. The ammonia is then utilised by the intestinal bacteria. This process means that nitrogenous waste products are excreted in faecal matter, rather than in urine, by the kidneys. However, if there are alterations in the gut microbiota, a dysbiosis, these can contribute to CKD progression and its associated complications. This is due to the production of uremic toxins by gut bacteria, which can lead to increased kidney damage and systemic inflammation.

- Uremic Toxin Production:
  Gut bacteria can metabolise dietary components and other substances, producing uremic toxins like indoxyl sulphate and *p*-cresyl sulphate. These

toxins accumulate in the bloodstream of individuals with CKD due to reduced kidney function, contributing to renal dysfunction.

- Dysbiosis and Increased Permeability:
  In CKD, the gut microbiota becomes dysbiotic, characterised by reduced diversity and altered composition of bacterial species. This dysbiosis can lead to increased intestinal permeability, allowing uremic toxins and other harmful substances to leak into the bloodstream, further exacerbating renal damage.
- Impact on Kidney Function:
  The accumulation of uremic toxins and the disruption of the intestinal barrier function can directly impair kidney function, contributing to the progression of CKD.
- Systemic Inflammation:
  Dysbiosis and the leakage of toxins can trigger a systemic inflammatory response, further contributing to kidney damage and other complications associated with CKD.
- Potential Therapeutic Targets:
  Understanding the role of the gut microbiome in CKD has opened avenues for potential therapeutic interventions, such as dietary modifications, prebiotic/probiotic supplementation and faecal microbiota transplantation (FMT).

In essence, the gut microbiome is not just a component of the digestive system; it is a vital player in overall health, including kidney health, and its dysbiosis can have significant consequences for renal function. Ensuring that the renal diet has good prebiotic fibre sources that support the biome, helping to prevent dysbiosis, is vital.

Vitamins and Minerals

Phosphate binders for dogs are supplements mixed into food to manage high phosphorus levels (hyperphosphatemia), commonly caused by kidney disease. They work directly in the gastrointestinal tract, binding to dietary phosphorus and forming an insoluble complex that is passed in the faeces rather than being absorbed into the blood.

Phosphate binders act as a 'magnet' or 'sponge' in the stomach/intestines, binding to dietary phosphate and preventing its absorption. These binders (irrespective of which is administered) must be given with food to be effective. They are ineffective if given without food, as they cannot bind to food phosphorus. If the animal refuses to eat the food with the binder mixed in, it can be administered immediately afterwards. The daily overall dose of the binder should be split between the number of meals that are given.

Common binders include calcium carbonate (blood calcium levels also need to be monitored), aluminium hydroxide or chitosan, often used when diet alone doesn't control phosphorus levels. Phosphate binders can be used with or without veterinary clinical renal (restricted phosphate diets) (Figure 18.1).

Within this study, those animals receiving Group 3 diets lived for a statistically significantly longer time. Table 18.2 shows that the diet used in Group 3 had significantly higher levels of essential fatty acids.

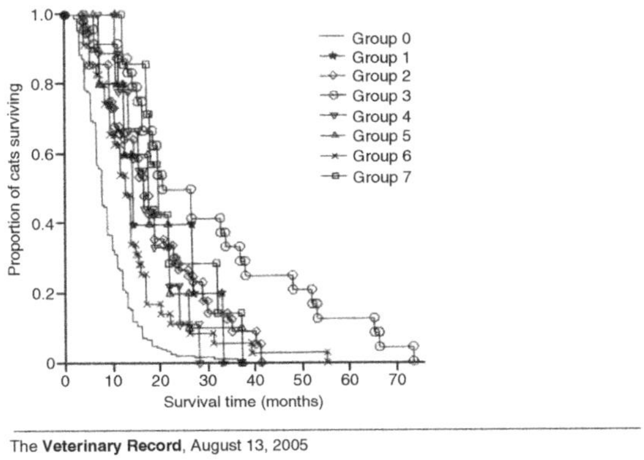

FIGURE 18.1 Shows survival curves for those animals on seven different types of renal diets. Ref. [4] / with permission of John Wiley & Sons.

TABLE 18.2 Composition of the seven brands of diets used within the study.

Diet	Type	Protein (g/MJ)	Phosphorus (g/MJ)	Sodium (g/MJ)	Potassium (g/MJ)	AA (g/MJ)	EPA (g/MJ)	Base excess[a] (mmol/kg DM)
1	Wet	12.6	0.20	0.13	0.48	0.25	0.05	168
2	Dry	13.1	0.24	0.12	0.42	0.03	ND	61
3	Wet	12.6	0.19	0.08	0.60	0.18	0.47	46
4	Dry	12.7	0.22	0.09	0.67	0.03	0.02	32
5	Dry	14.9	0.34	0.21	0.57	0.06	0.11	154
6	Wet	11.8	0.17	0.10	0.40	0.14	ND	35
7	Dry	12.8	0.21	0.11	0.49	0.02	ND	48

[a] Base excess was calculated according to Kienzle and others [7]. Data derived from Plantinga and Beynen [8].
AA, arachidonic acid; EPA, eicosapentaenoic acid; DM, dry matter; ND, not detected.
Diet 3 showed the longest survival curves within the groups.

Animals with renal insufficiency have a reduced ability to maintain hydration levels. Due to polyuria, water-soluble vitamins and electrolytes are also lost. Vitamin B12 is an important factor in the control of appetite and is often deficient in renal patients. Oral supplementation is required; this can be easily achieved through an enriched diet or supplements.

REFERENCES

1. Groves, E. (2019). Nutrition in senior cats and dogs: how does the diet need to change, when and why? *Companion Animal* 24 (2): 91.
2. Sparkes, A.H., Caney, S., Chalhoub, S. et al. (2016). ISFM consensus guidelines on the diagnosis and management of feline chronic kidney disease. *J. Feline Med. Surg.* 18: 219.
3. Taylor, E.J., Adams, C., and Neville, R. (1995). Some nutritional aspects of ageing in dogs and cats. *Proc. Nutr. Soc.* 54: 645.

4. Plantinga, E.A., Everts, H., Kastelein, A.M.C., and Beynen, A.C. (2005). Retrospective study of the survival of cats with acquired chronic renal insufficiency offered different commercial diets. *Vet. Rec.* 157: 185.
5. Pekel, A.Y., Mülazımoğlu, S.B., and Acar, N. (2020). Taste preferences and diet palatability in cats. *J. Appl. Anim. Res.* 48 (1): 281.
6. Cupp, C., Kerr, W.W., Patil, A.R. et al. (2008). The role of nutritional interventions in the longevity and maintenance of long-term health in aging cats. *Int. J. Appl. Res. Vet. Med.* 6 (2): 69.
7. Kienzle, E., Schuknecht, A., and Meyer, H. (1991). Influence of food composition on the urine pH in cats. *J. Nutr.* 121: S87–S88.
8. Plantinga, E.A. and Beynen, A.C. (2004). Vergelijkende analyse van commerciële nierdiëten voor katten, met bijzondere aandacht voor de vetzuursamenstelling. *Tijdschrift voor Diergeneeskunde* 129: 656–662.

CHAPTER 19

Urinary System

CANINE UROLITHIASIS

Urolithiasis in dogs can be a complex, multifactorial disorder and may require different approaches to aid in the recurrence of crystals and stones. Careful identification of the urolith present is needed to make the best judgement regarding the type of management, surgical or medical. Medical management is based on the diet for the animal. Each urolith will have optimum management, but a compromise may be required, as many uroliths can be comprised of a combination of different minerals. Careful monitoring throughout is needed.

Urolithiasis is considered to be a common disorder of the urinary tract in dogs [1]. Different breeds are more highly represented for certain uroliths than others. Breeds found to be significantly overrepresented for calcium oxalate uroliths included the Chihuahua, Miniature Poodle and Yorkshire Terrier. Staffordshire bull terriers and English bulldogs were at increased risk for cystine uroliths [2].

Clinical signs of urolithiasis may be the first indication of an underlying systemic disorder or a defect in the structure or function of the urinary tract. As with feline idiopathic cystitis (FIC), urolithiasis shouldn't be viewed as a single disease process but rather as a sequel of underlying abnormalities. Examination of the urolith composition will aid in determining the aetiology. A full dietary history is required, along with blood serum biochemistry and urinalysis of the concentration of calculogenic minerals, crystallisation promoters and crystallisation inhibitors. Urinary diets for dogs (and cats) can be divided into those that promote dissolution through changing the pH of the urine and those that act by diluting the concentration of the urine. In all cases, dietary management should only commence once obstruction (if present) has been resolved.

NUTRITIONAL MANAGEMENT

Canine urolithiasis is a disorder that needs close monitoring long term due to the nature of the reformation of crystals and stones. Dissolution and prevention of any future stones and crystals is the main aim of long-term management, and this can be achieved by several means that can be monitored by veterinary nurses within a clinic setting. The other main aims are to:

- Decrease the amount of calculogenic materials within the urine.
- Increase water intake and frequency of urination.
- Promote an optimal pH; this is dependent on the urolith present.
- Help the animal obtain its ideal weight and body condition score (BCS).
- Perform regular urine and blood sampling and ensure compliance from the owner.
- Owner education in preventative measures.

Where dissolution of uroliths is possible with medical management (Table 19.1), this should be instigated rather than surgical intervention. There are several reasons for this; not all stones and crystals will be removed during a cystotomy, and suture material can act as a nidus for further urolith formation. Calcium oxalate uroliths cannot be medically managed and will need surgical intervention.

CLINICAL NUTRITION

The nutrition recommended can alter slightly depending on the stone or crystal present, and therefore, any clinical nutritional recommendations for specific stones are discussed separately. The consumption of water, however, is the same no matter which is present (Figure 19.1).

TABLE 19.1 Urolith formations and treatments, with urinary pH preferences.

Type of urolith	Urinary pH during formation	Target urinary pH	Treatment
Struvite	Alkaline	5.9–6.3	Calculolytic diet or surgical removal
Calcium oxalate	Variable but usually acidic	7.1–7.7	Surgical removal
Ammonium urate	Acidic	7.1–7.7	Calculolytic diet and allopurinol
Cystine	Acidic	7.1–7.7	Calculolytic diet or surgical removal
Silicate	Usually acidic	7.1–7.7	Surgical removal

Adapted from Ref. [2].

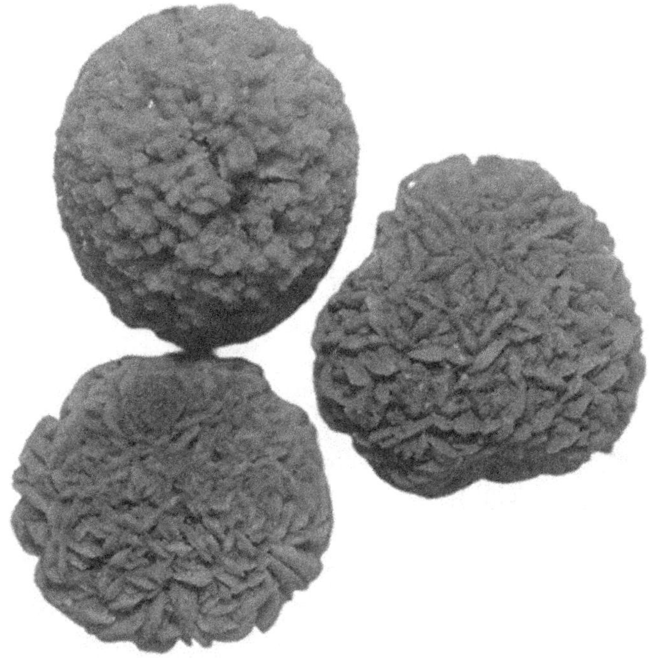

FIGURE 19.1 Calcium oxalate stones need to be surgically removed. dinu_rj/Shutterstock.

Water

Water intake is a vital factor in dogs with, or those that have a predisposition to, canine urolithiasis. The solute load of the diet influences total water intake by a large factor, the same as with cats. The use of a moist diet can aid in increasing water consumption in some dogs that don't drink enough. Adding additional water to the diet can be useful in some cases, but it can alter the palatability of the diet for some. Encouragement to increase the consumption of water can also be achieved by increasing access by placing more bowls of water around the dog's environment. Use of bottled, pre-boiled water or water that has been left to stand will have little or no chlorine that can be detected by the dog. Some dogs will also play with/eat ice cubes, which is especially useful in warm weather, or drink flavoured water. Fruit juices can be good; meat/broths can contain minerals and salts. Their use depends on the type of uroliths present, see Box 19.1.

Increases in water consumption will increase the total volume of urine produced. Crystals precipitate out into the urine when supersaturation occurs. Urine becomes saturated when the salt content completely dissolves within the fluid. Any additional salt or decrease in the relative fluid volume will result in precipitation of the salts in urine at this stage, which is said to be supersaturated. Supersaturation of the urine is the initial stage of crystal urolith formation (Figure 19.2). Although urine supersaturation is fundamental for orthogenesis, the whole process is complex and multifactorial [1]. Veterinary professionals recommended that the animal's urine should remain

Box 19.1 Foods with a low, medium or high purine content

The following foods are low in purine:

- Eggs, nuts and peanut butter
- Low-fat and fat-free cheese and ice cream
- Skim or 1% milk
- Soup made without meat extract or broth
- Vegetables that are not on the medium-purine list below
- All fruit and fruit juices
- Bread, pasta, rice, cake, cornbread and popcorn
- Water, soda, tea, coffee and cocoa
- Sugar, sweets and gelatine
- Fat and oil

Medium-purine foods:

- **Meats:** Limit the following to 100–150 g (4–6 oz) each day
  - Meat and poultry
  - Crab, lobster, oysters and shrimp
- **Vegetables:** Limit the following vegetables to ½ cup each day
  - Asparagus
  - Cauliflower
  - Spinach
  - Mushrooms
  - Green peas
- Beans, peas and lentils
- Oats and oatmeal
- Wheat germ and bran

High-purine foods:

- Limit or avoid foods high in purine
- Anchovies, sardines, scallops and mussels
- Tuna, codfish, herring and haddock
- Wild game meats, like goose and duck
- Organ meats, such as brains, heart, kidney, liver and sweetbreads
- Gravies and sauces made with meat
- Yeast extracts taken in the form of a supplement

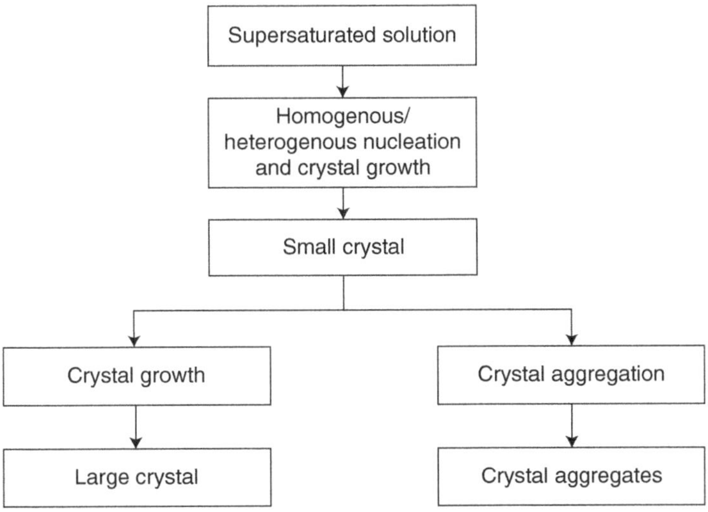

FIGURE 19.2 Supersaturation leads to crystal growth and aggregation.

dilute and have no strong smell. Bitch's urine does bleach/kill the grass where urination commonly occurs. This doesn't reflect that crystals or uroliths are present. The use of filtered water in hard water areas can aid in reducing the intake of minerals, such as calcium carbonate, which is found in hard water areas. Many small-breed dogs will urinate less frequently than larger-breed dogs [3]. These breeds do need to be taken out more often to urinate. Access to the garden where the door is left open or a dog flap may not ensure that the dog is urinating more frequently, and supervising the dog and giving the command to urinate may be more beneficial [4].

Urate Urolithiasis

Dalmatians have a high risk factor for recurrent urate uroliths (Figure 19.3), high enough that prophylactic therapy should be actively considered for this breed. Some texts state that Dalmatians are more susceptible as they lack the enzyme uricase, which

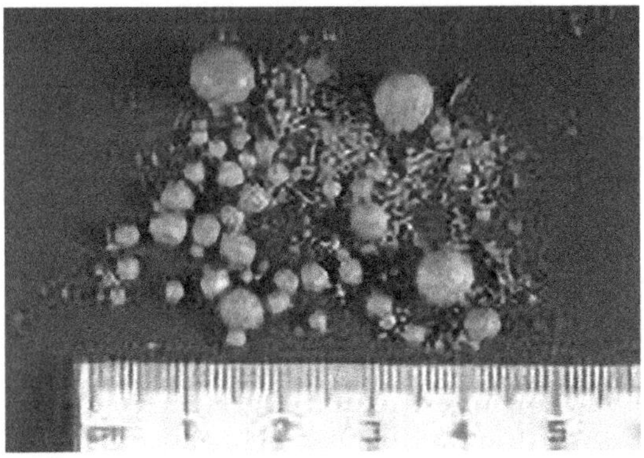

FIGURE 19.3 Uric acid stones. Vetstream Ltd / https://www.vetlexicon.com/canis/urinary/images/urolithiasis-ammonium-urate-and-uric-acid-stones/ / last accessed on July 11, 2025

converts uric acid to allantoin. Their urine, therefore, contains higher levels of urates than other breeds [5]. In other texts [6, 7], uric acid metabolism is not caused by the absence of hepatic uricase. With uricase enzyme levels being comparable to those in other breeds. The cause has been attributed to the impaired transport of uric acid into the hepatocytes, which may reduce the rate of hepatic oxidation. Another factor can be attributed to the proximal renal tubules of Dalmatians reabsorbing less and secreting more urate than the kidneys of other breeds of dogs [6].

The nutrition aims of dietary management of urate urolithiasis include:

- Restricting the protein level.
- Increasing the source of non-protein calories.
- Promoting an alkaline urine pH.

Clinical Nutrition

Proteins

The protein levels in a diet designed to aid in urate urolithiasis can have overall restricted levels of proteins (1.6–2.2 g protein/100 kcal metabolisable energy [ME]) [7]. Especially those proteins which contain larger amounts of nucleic acids, as they contain purines, for example, protein from muscle or organ tissues. Milk proteins (casein) and eggs provide a suitable source, as they contain a lower amount of purines but also have a high biological value, which is required when a restriction on protein levels is required in the diet. Box 19.1 gives a list of different foods that are high, medium and low in purine content.

Allopurinol is a xanthine oxidase inhibitor, which reduces the rate of urate excretion into the urine. It decreases the production of uric acid by inhibiting the conversion of hypoxanthine to xanthine and xanthine to uric acid. Allopurinol does need to be added to the diet when dissolution of urate uroliths is required, though checking the dietary manufacturers' guidelines is recommended.

Carbohydrates and Fats

Due to the restriction in protein levels, there must be a sufficient supply of non-protein calories. A higher-than-normal fat content can arise from this (20% DMB), and care should be given to the weight control of the animal. The level of fats also aids in obtaining the preferred urine pH.

Vitamins and Minerals

As with any disease or disorder whose clinical symptoms include polyuria, the water-soluble vitamins should be supplemented. With urolithiasis, however, vitamin C should not be supplemented as it is a precursor of oxalate and can predispose its formation.

The alkalising agent used in these diets is commonly potassium citrate and calcium carbonate. If the target urinary pH is not reached, then additional potassium citrate can be added to the diet at a starting dose rate of 50–100 mg/kg bodyweight (bwt) PO bid, the amount given to effect [7].

Struvite Uroliths

Struvite uroliths in dogs, as in cats, are the most commonly occurring uroliths in the United Kingdom and the United States [6]. Infection-induced struvite uroliths are common in dogs, and a positive culture result should prompt initiation of antimicrobial therapy alongside nutritional management. The bacteria present tend to be those that are urease-producing.

Nutritional aims of dietary management of struvite uroliths include:

- The dissolution of uroliths within the bladder.
- Prevent the formation of recurring uroliths or crystals.
- Promote an acidic urine pH.
- Increasing water intake and encouraging the dog to urinate more frequently.

Clinical Nutrition

Proteins

Restricted levels of protein are required (1.47 g protein/100 kcal ME) [1], but a high biological value is needed. When protein levels are this restricted, it is not advisable to feed this diet in the long term. The urine acidifying substance in diets designed for struvite dissolution is DL-methionine, used at a dose rate of 0.5 g/kg of diet [1].

Carbohydrates

The majority of calories obtained from the diet need to be obtained from a non-protein source. Thus, proportionately, the carbohydrate and fat levels of the ME are increased in these diets.

Fats

Struvite diets can have very high-fat levels (~26% dry matter (DM)), so much so that in some brands, only tinned formulas are available. Feeding diets with this high a fat content to dogs with hyperlipidaemia, pancreatitis or even at-risk groups (such as Schnauzers and Spaniels) is contraindicated.

Vitamins and Minerals

Decreased amounts of phosphorus (24 mg phosphorus/100 kcal ME) and magnesium (3.3 mg magnesium/100 kcal ME) are present in diets designed to aid urinary tract issues, as these are the constituents of the struvite urolith [1]. Sodium levels are often increased in these diets in order to increase water intake (23.3 mg sodium/100 kcal

ME). The use of the antioxidants vitamin E and beta-carotene is often supplemented, as it helps to reduce oxidative damage and helps to combat urolithiasis. As an oxalate precursor, vitamin C should not be supplemented when feeding diets designed for struvite dissolution.

Calcium Oxalate Uroliths

Calcium oxalate uroliths are the second most commonly occurring uroliths in the dog.

Nutritional aims of dietary management include:

- Promoting an alkaline urinary pH.
- Reducing the amounts of calcium, sodium and oxalates within the diet.
- Increase water consumption and the frequency of urination.

Clinical Nutrition

Protein

A low protein diet is required, with levels of 1.6–2.2 g/100 kcal ME have been suggested [7], in cases where calcium oxalate uroliths are present.

Fats and Carbohydrates

Non-protein calories are required in the diet to prevent protein catabolism. Thus, levels of fats and carbohydrates are higher than normal, for example, fat can be as high as 26% DMB and carbohydrates 60% DMB. Weight management can be a problem in dogs, which are predisposed to weight gain.

Vitamins and Minerals

Vitamins D and C should not be supplemented in the diet. Vitamin D increases the absorption of calcium from the diet, whereas vitamin C acts as a precursor to oxalates. The levels of calcium in the diet should be restricted, but not reduced, as with levels of sodium. Restricted calcium levels are approximately 0.68% DMB. Sodium increases calcium excretion into the urine, and a dietary level of 0.1–0.2% sodium DMB or 45–55 mg sodium/100 kcal ME is recommended [7]. The digestibility of the diet and the individual's absorption ability of vitamins and minerals will vary greatly, and thus, monitoring of levels may be required.

Cystine Urolithiasis

Cystine uroliths are uncommon in both cats and dogs but arise due to a metabolic defect where the reabsorption of filtered cystine in the proximal tubule is impaired [8]. Once in the urine, cystine is very insoluble, especially in acidic urine.

Nutritional aims in the management of cystine uroliths include:

- Promoting an alkaline urine pH.
- Reducing the amount of cystine produced by the body.
- Increase water consumption and frequency of urination.

Clinical Nutrition

Protein

A low protein diet is required (9–11% protein DM), as this will aid in the reduction of the total daily excretion of cystine [1].

Carbohydrates and Fats

Due to the low levels of protein in the diet, calories have to be obtained from these nutrients. Care should be taken with diets that are high in fats, similar to that described in a diet designed for struvite uroliths.

Vitamins and Minerals

Low sodium levels are also required, as sodium excretion can enhance cystine excretion. Low sodium in combination with low protein levels tends to increase the urine volume, which further decreases the urinary concentration of cystine [7]. To create an alkaline urine pH, supplementation with potassium citrate (50–100 mg/kg bwt PO bid) is required.

Silicate Uroliths

These uroliths are more commonly seen in male dogs (96%) than in females (4%) [1]. Most likely due to females being able to pass smaller uroliths before they can induce clinical signs. Foods which contain large amounts of plant-derived materials are thought to be a predisposing factor for silicate uroliths. Another factor being the consumption of soil, as silica in the soil passes through to the plants and is readily absorbed via the intestines.

Dietary management of dogs suffering from silicate uroliths is for prevention. A change of diet to one which doesn't contain large amounts of plant-derived materials and increases the volume of urine produced are the main factors. A debate has arisen regarding the urinary pH levels; alkalisation of the urine to increase the solubility of silica is unknown [9].

Feeding a Dog with Urolithiasis

Nearly all diets aimed at dissolution or prevention of uroliths are potentially higher in fat levels, mainly due to the requirement for non-protein calories. Care should be given when transferring a dog to these diets. Caution should also be given to those dogs which are likely to gain weight, or those, which are predisposed to hyperlipidaemia or pancreatitis. Diarrhoea can occur when high-fat levels are fed, and a combination with a high-fibre diet, which is aimed at urolith prevention, may be required.

Calculolytic diets are only successful when fed alone. The addition of treats and home-cooked foods can undo the desired effect of the diet. It is equally important that the urolith analysis is correct. Stones, which are of mixed composition, are difficult to dissolve, and surgical removal may be the treatment of choice. In dogs suffering from struvite urolithiasis, if you have the suspicion that additional snacks or treats are being fed, a blood sample analysis can be useful. In dogs being fed certain veterinary struvite dissolution diets, a low plasma urea concentration of less than 4 mmol/l (BUN 10 mg/dl) is found [1]. Above these levels suggests additional feeding.

Monitoring of dogs suffering from urolithiasis is vital, including body weight and body condition. A full nutritional assessment should be performed on every pet at every visit [10]. Urinalysis should be performed at least every six months once dissolution has occurred. Preventative measures involve feeding a diet which promotes the correct urine pH, promotes undersaturation of the urine, provides calories from a non-protein source and is relatively low in salts that are the building blocks for the uroliths that the animal suffers from.

CONCLUSION

Dogs that have suffered from any form of urolithiasis need to have regular urinalysis whilst on the diet, including pH and microscopy performed. Client education can be key in prevention for at-risk breeds and those that are over their ideal BCS. This includes increasing water intake as much as possible in all groups and the frequency of urination.

FELINE LOWER URINARY TRACT DISEASE

Urine is a composite of a complex solution of both organic and inorganic ions. Crystals can grow and form when an imbalance occurs in this complex solution. These reasons include diet, decreased water consumption, urine pH alterations or a relative lack of inhibitors of crystallisation [1].

Dietary manipulation can aid in reducing the risk factors of formation and help with dissolution. However, there are many other factors that need to be taken into consideration and addressed during the overall management. These include:

- Take a full history of the environmental factors and give advice regarding these factors. Discuss strategies to reduce stressors for the cat.
- Increasing the solubility of the minerals. This is achieved by obtaining an optimal urinary pH or reducing urine specific gravity, which will dissolve any crystals and aid in the prevention of any further formation.
- Eliminate or reduce the risk of supersaturation by increasing overall urine volume.

- Increase the presence of inhibitors of crystallisation.
- Use of an appropriate diet to aid the animal in obtaining and maintaining an ideal BCS if required.

Diets That Alter Urinary pH

Struvite crystals are commonly seen in cats suffering from FLUTD or urethral obstructions. If urinary pH adaptation is being utilised for dissolution, the pH needs to be neutral to acidic, as the crystals form in an alkaline environment. A range of 5.9 to 6.1 is ideal for dissolution, whereas 6.2 to 6.4 is recommended for prevention. The average urinary pH of a domestic cat consuming a natural diet (small rodents) is pH 6.3. Cats receiving long-term dietary acidifiers (phosphoric acid and ammonium chloride acidifiers) can suffer from a transient negative potassium balance. Long-term potassium depletion will stimulate ammonia synthesis at the same site as chronic metabolic acidosis. Acidifying therapeutic veterinary diets need to have potassium levels higher than the NRC minimum allowance of 0.6% (DMB) [8]. The use of urinary acidifiers alongside an acidifying food is not recommended, as it can lead to metabolic acidosis. The alterations in pH may increase the solubility of some of the solutes within the urine and, in some cases, decrease the solubility of others. This complex and competing interplay between nutritional requirements of the management of oxalate and struvite urolithiasis requires a careful selection in the long-term dietary control of FLUTD.

Differences in the nutritional management of cats suffering from oxalate crystals include obtaining a less acidic urinary pH of 6.6–6.8. Citrate can be supplemented in diets specifically for cats suffering from oxalate crystals or uroliths. The citrate increases the urinary pH and forms soluble complexes with the calcium to inhibit calcium oxalate formation.

Diets That Alter Solute Load/Water Intake

Water intake is a vital factor in cats especially those with a predisposition to FLUTD, as increases in water consumption will increase the total volume of urine produced. The solute load of the diet influences total water intake by a large factor. Use of a moist diet might be preferred, and additional water can also be mixed in if required, but use of specific clinical urinary diets that are designed to reduce supersaturation of the urine and increase water intake have been shown to be as effective in dry formulations as the wet. Encouragement to increase the consumption of water can also be achieved by increasing access and the number of bowls. Preferences for the type and size of water bowls need to be considered. Cats can be deterred from drinking fresh tap water due to the chlorine content. Use of bottled, pre-boiled water, or water that has been left to stand will have little or no chlorine that can be detected by the cat.

Urine becomes saturated when the salt content is completely dissolved within the fluid. Any additional salt or decrease in the relative fluid volume will result in precipitation of the salts. Urine at this stage is said to be supersaturated, and crystals will precipitate out into the urine. Supersaturation of the urine is the initial stage of crystal urolith formation. Although urine supersaturation is fundamental for urthogenesis, the whole process is a complex and multifactorial.

Protein

Excessive levels of protein need to be avoided in cases where struvite crystals and alkaline urine are present. High protein levels can influence pH; a prime example of this is the difference in urine pH between cats and dogs. Cats have higher protein consumption than dogs and, therefore, an increased urinary pH. Increasing the protein level in the diet also increases urinary calcium excretion, uric acid and oxalate excretion. Excess dietary protein should be avoided by feeding a food that contains 30–45% DM protein [8].

Fats

Diets that promote urinary tract health do tend to have a higher fat content. This is due to the increased energy density, which overall reduces mineral intake. When metabolised, fat produces the highest metabolic water contribution, which also benefits the animal. Due to the increased fat content, some veterinary clinical diets are not available in a dry form. Obesity is a major risk factor of FLUTD. Nutritional assessment of BCS, and if overweight, use of a lower-calorie urinary diet would be beneficial.

Vitamins and Minerals

Struvite precipitates form when the urine becomes supersaturated with magnesium, anionic phosphate and ammonium. Therapeutic diets avoid excess dietary magnesium, but low urinary magnesium concentrations have the potential to increase the risk of the formation of calcium-containing uroliths. The intake of magnesium and calcium also influences urinary phosphate concentrations. Highlighting the importance of regular urinalysis when on a therapeutic urinary diet.

The addition of sodium to the diet is occasionally utilised to aid in the increase of water intake. Increasing the salt content of the diet can aid in diuresis and lower the urine specific gravity. Sodium, however, does increase calcium excretion into the urine. Excessive sodium levels are also discouraged in older animals due to the possibility of decreased renal function. A sodium level of 1.2% (DMB) has proven to present a health risk to cats when being fed this level in the long term [9]. Adding antioxidants can help combat urolithiasis by reducing oxidative cell damage.

Supplements

The use of nutraceuticals in cases of FLUTD is commonplace. Glycosaminoglycans (GAGs) and chondroitin are widely used to provide a protective lining to the bladder. In the healthy animal, there is a GAG layer that lines the urothelium in the bladder and contributes towards the protection of the bladder wall from substances (e.g. crystals) present within the urine. Cats suffering from FLUTD can have a decreased excretion of urinary GAGs, and deficiencies in the GAG layer can contribute to urothelial damage, ulceration and inflammation of the bladder wall [9]. These types of nutraceuticals do not prevent the reoccurrence of the crystals but aid in the reoccurrence of some of the clinical signs. Evaluation of treatment effectiveness should be made over a sufficient period (e.g. three to six months). There is the potential for placebo effect as stress and anxiety within the household can play a significant impact into recurrence of FLUTD.

Feeding a Cat with FLUTD

Free-choice feeding is preferable in cats, this is when a controlled known volume of diet is offered daily and the animal has free choice of when it is to be consumed. This scenario might not be possible if the cat is within a multi-pet household. When any animal consumes food, gastric acid is secreted and creates a temporary net acid loss from the body and alkalisation of the urine. This is referred to as the postprandial alkaline tide. The alkaline tide is caused by the secretion of bicarbonate into the blood by parietal cells of the stomach. A transient bicarbonisation is produced, and an increase in urinary pH. Acidifiers in the diet will offset this increase in pH. If the diet is offered free choice, the cat will eat little and often. These feeding habits result in a smaller but more prolonged alkaline tide. This can reduce the likelihood of struvite precipitate formation.

Recommendations should be given to clients about preventative measures in all cats. There are clear risk factors associated with FLUTD, some of which cannot be helped (i.e. age, breed and gender) and others, such as lifestyle and obesity, which can. Neutering does play a significant impact on the risk of bladder stones (the risk of oxalate increasing sevenfold and the risk of struvite 3.5-fold) [11]. Educating the owner to ensure an adequate water intake and limiting weight gain post-neutering is vital.

REDUCING STRESS IN CATS

The influence of behavioural responses in the cat has been widely linked to the occurrence of FLUTD in cats. Clients need to be made aware of this link and given appropriate advice to help their cat. Many cats can be presented to the veterinary practice for behavioural problems with inappropriate urination, but FLUTD needs to be ruled out prior to instigation of behavioural treatments.

- Food intake disorders (anorexia or overfeeding).
- Overgrooming (bald areas) or under-grooming (matted or soiled fur).
- House soiling, inappropriate urination or defecation.
- Decreasing levels of activity, increased rest or feigned sleep.
- Appearing withdrawn (reduced desire to play or interact), hiding.
- Extreme vigilance and heightened startle response.

- Defensive aggression towards people and other cats in the household, for example, hissing.
- Increased dependency or social withdrawal (dependent on personality type).
- Changes in patterns of behaviour, for example, spending a more significant amount of time indoors, irrespective of normal seasonal changes.
- Urine spraying.

Helping the client to understand these sometimes very subtle signs can be very difficult for clients. In multi-cat households, the presence of other cats can be the main cause, and removal of the cause is impossible. Owners need to be supported to make changes to the household to help the stressed family member. Dietary transitions are classed as a stressor in cats, especially when changing the texture of the diet. There needs to be sufficient resources in the household to reduce competition for them. This means that more litter trays, food bowls and water bowls are required than cats within the household. All these resources need to be separate from one another, as cats do not like to eat, drink or eliminate in the same area.

Key Points

- Increase water intake and thus urinary dilution. Urine specific gravity is a more important factor than urine pH.
- Perform regular urinalysis, even once dissolution has been achieved. It should also be recommended that a full blood haematology and biochemistry test be performed on a regular basis.
- Educate clients to take preventative measures against the formation of urinary calculi throughout a cat's life, starting from a young age.

REFERENCES

1. Osborne, C.A., Bartges, J.W., Lulich, J.P. et al. (2000). Canine urolithiasis. In: *Small Animal Clinical Nutrition*, 4e (ed. M.S. Hand, C.D. Thatcher, R.L. Remillard, and P. Roudebush), 605–688. Missouri: Mark Morris Institute.
2. Roe, K., Pratt, A., Lulich, J. et al. (2012). Analysis of 14,008 uroliths from dogs in the UK over a 10-year period. *J. Small Anim. Pract.* 53: 634–640.
3. Stevenson, A.E. and Markwell, P.J. (2001). Comparison of urine composition of healthy Labrador retrievers and miniature schnauzers. *Am. J. Vet. Res.* 62: 1782–1786.
4. Perea, S.C. (2009). Nutritional management of urolithiasis. *NAVC Clinician's Brief* 47–50.
5. Agar, S. (2001). *Small Animal Nutrition*. Edinburgh: Butterworth Heinemann.
6. Buffington, T., Holloway, C., and Abood, S. (2004). *Manual of Veterinary Dietetics*. Missouri: Elsevier Saunders.
7. Senior, D.F. (1996). Urolithiasis – a nutritional perspective. In: *BSAVA Manual of Companion Animal Nutrition and Feeding* (ed. N. Kelly and J. Wills), 188–197. Gloucester: BSAVA Publications.

8. Bovee, K.C. (1984). Genetic and metabolic diseases of the kidney. In: *Canine Nephrology* (ed. K.C. Bovee), 339–354. Pennsylvania: Harwell Publications.
9. Osborne, C.A., Clinton, C.W., Kim, K.M., and Mansfield, C.F. (1986). Etiopathogenesis, clinical manifestations and management of canine silica urolithiasis. *Vet. Clin. North Am. Small Anim. Pract.* 16: 185–207.
10. Freeman, L., Becvarova, I., Cave, N., MacKay, C., Nguyen, P., Rama, B., Takashima, G., Tiffin, R., Tsjimoto, H., & van Beukelen, P. (2011). WSAVA nutritional assessment guidelines. *J. Small Anim. Pract.* 52 (7): 385–396. https://doi.org/https://doi.org/10.1111/j.1748-5827.2011.01079.x
11. Okafor, C. C., Pearl, D. L., Lefebvre, S. L., Wang, M., Yang, M., Blois, S. L., Lund, E. M., & Dewey, C. E. (2013). Risk factors associated with struvite urolithiasis in dogs evaluated at general care veterinary hospitals in the United States. *J. Am. Vet. Med. Assoc.*, 243 (12): 1737–1745. https://doi.org/https://doi.org/10.2460/javma.243.12.1737

CHAPTER 20

Pancreatitis

There are many scenarios in practice where animals present with acute, chronic and acute-on-chronic bouts of pancreatitis. By investigating the cause of pancreatitis, possibilities include an association with being fed high-fat diets and dietary indiscretions; in a clinical setting, dietary manipulation could be instigated to reduce the risk of pancreatitis or the risk of reoccurrence.

Many animals are placed on low-fat diets when diagnosed with pancreatitis. Nutritional recommendations for adult dogs are a minimum of 5.5 g/100 g dry matter of the food consumed, based on an energy requirement of 95 kcal/kg bwt$^{0.75}$. There is no recommendation on the type of fats, but the essential fatty acids are provided.

When reviewing pancreatitis (whether acute bouts or chronic disease), there is often reference made to high-fat diets being a predisposing factor to pancreatitis and that the treatment regimen includes feeding a low-fat diet. Discussion in clinical practice suggests that high-fat diets lead to persistent hyperlipidaemia (whether high cholesterol, lipids or triglycerides), which predisposes to pancreatitis. Many texts refer to hyperlipidaemia being shown to be a predisposition to the clinical signs associated with pancreatitis, but on examination of many of these texts, they have been misquoted, with hyperlipidaemia not being quoted as a proven predisposition. The cited research papers, Haig [1] and Yago et al. [2], showed that high-fat diets were fed, and there was an association with an increase in pancreatic secretion and the enzymes within the secretions, but no correlation with clinical signs.

IS FEEDING A HIGH-FAT DIET A PREDISPOSING FACTOR TO PANCREATITIS IN DOGS?

In the first-opinion veterinary practice, we are often told not to feed high-fat diets to dogs with, or predisposed to, pancreatitis. This includes those with hyperlipidaemia, even without clinical signs of pancreatitis, as there is a high incidence of inducing an acute pancreatitis bout.

PREDISPOSING FACTORS TO PANCREATITIS

Pancreatitis is a very common disease in both the dog and the cat, with the potential for very serious consequences [3]. The clinical picture of dogs and cats with pancreatitis varies greatly (from very mild to severe or even fatal) [4], which highlights the importance of removing avoidable risk factors. Predisposing factors to chronic pancreatitis include a breed disposition for Cocker Spaniels, Cavalier King Charles Spaniels, Border Collies and Boxers in UK-based studies [5]. In the same study, Cocker Spaniels had an increased relative risk for both acute and chronic combined. Research into English Cocker Spaniels suggests it is part of a polysystemic immune-mediated disease in this breed [6]. The histological and clinical appearance is different in different breeds, suggesting that aetiologies may also be different. Overweight and obesity increase incidence rates [7], as does neutering [8] and hyperlipidaemia [9]. Certain medications such as phenobarbitone in combination with potassium bromide [10], azathioprine (though a very small-scale study with concurrent use of prednisolone) [11] and many more beyond the scope of this literature review, have all been shown to increase risk. Many of these predisposing factors are potentially cause and effect, and there have been proven links between many of them: obesity and breed, obesity and neutering and hyperlipidaemia (including hypertriglyceridaemia) and obesity [12]. Breed, neuter status and age are risk factors that can't be altered, but body condition score (overweight or obese) and diet can be controlled.

There is emerging work investigating serum calcium levels in acute pancreatitis cases. They have been shown to have decreased 25-(OH)D levels compared to healthy individuals, which the authors postulated might be associated with calcium imbalances and mortality rate in canine acute pancreatitis [13]. There were limitations of the study (number in the study and no histological evaluation of the pancreas), but as a pilot study, it showed that there are some very interesting areas of study that also showed associated alterations in C-reactive protein (CRP), a marker of inflammation, with the vitamin D and calcium imbalances and the possibility of monitoring potential risk factors [13]. With vitamin D being a fat-soluble vitamin, there is also a postulated link between fat content and vitamin levels [13].

The exact mechanism of inducing acute pancreatitis is unclear, but it is thought to be due to increased levels of chylomicrons in the bloodstream. Chylomicrons are usually formed one to three hours postprandially and cleared within eight hours. However, when triglyceride levels exceed 1,000 mg/dl, chylomicrons are almost always present. These low-density particles are very large and may obstruct capillaries, leading to local ischaemia and acidaemia. The degradation of triglycerides, by pancreatic lipase, to free fatty acids can lead to cytotoxic injury, resulting in further local injury that causes positive feedback to increase inflammatory mediators and free radicals, thus instigating pancreatitis [14].

Canines, however, exhibit unique characteristics in lipid metabolism, allowing hyperlipidaemia to be subdivided into two categories, based on whether irregularities are occurring in exogenous (lipid-rich diets) and/or endogenous lipid metabolism pathways [15]. Incidence rates of hyperlipidaemia in canines are not often quoted, just stated as being common [4, 16, 17]. Incidence rates in asymptomatic Schnauzers and Shetland Sheepdogs found that the frequency of primary hyperlipidaemia was between 32.8% and 56.4% [16]. The pathogenesis of hypertriglyceridemia-induced pancreatitis is poorly understood [3]. It is postulated that pancreatic lipase might break down triglycerides to fatty acids within the pancreas, resulting in acinar damage [18]. The pancreatic acinar cell is the functional unit of the exocrine pancreas. It synthesises, stores and secretes digestive enzymes. Inappropriate early activation of trypsin within the acinar cells activates other zymogens and causes auto-digestion and severe inflammation [3]. An alternative theory in the same paper suggested that hyperviscosity (due to increased lipid content) of the blood can compromise pancreatic oxygen supply [18].

Watson et al. [19] investigated various clinical parameters of 61 dogs presented to a veterinary teaching hospital between 2002 and 2006. The published report of the work noted that the dogs had a perceived reduction of abdominal pain when fed a low-fat diet. Though there was no quantitative measurement of pain scores in these animals with no control diet. The study doesn't state the nutrient composition of the food or the type of fat that the diet contained. In this study, all of the cases were naturally occurring rather than induced pancreatitis, with multiple different breeds and cross-breeds. No statistical analysis was conducted as there was no control group, and specificity, positive and negative predictive values also could not be calculated. There was discussion in the paper that obese dogs (body condition score 5/5) had a higher predisposition to pancreatitis; there was no discussion regarding what these dogs were being fed or whether the dogs with the higher BCS had a higher rate of hyperlipidaemia.

Lem et al. [7] specifically looked at dietary factors and links with pancreatitis. Various continuous data (age, weight, hospitalisation time, number of days receiving fluids via IV and serum cPLI) were statistically analysed using the Kolmogorov-Smirnov test to see whether there was a normal distribution – which there wasn't. Due to these results being summarised as median and range, the Mann–Whitney U test was used to compare values between case and control dogs. It should be noted that the control dogs were those diagnosed with renal failure, as the number of animals that are presented to the hospital with renal disease is similar to that of being diagnosed with pancreatitis. Statistical analysis for the dietary factors was summarised as frequencies and compared between the case and control groups by the use of $\chi 2$ or Fisher's exact test. The crude odds ratios (ORs), 95% confidence intervals (CIs) and Pearson $\chi 2$ p values were calculated. Adjusted ORs, 95% CIs and Mantel–Haenszel $\chi 2$ p values were calculated after stratification based on disease severity. Based on the information extracted from the clinical history, ingesting an unusual food item (OR, 4.3) increased the odds of pancreatitis compared to the control group, so those that ate an unusual food item were 4.3 times more likely to develop pancreatitis than those that didn't. Based on information gathered through a telephone questionnaire, ingesting unusual food items (OR, 6.1), ingesting table scraps the week before diagnosis (OR, 2.2) or throughout life (OR, 2.2), and getting into the dustbin/rubbish (OR, 13.2) increased the odds of pancreatitis, compared to the control group. Multivariable modelling indicated that reporting exposure to ≥ 1 dietary factor during the telephone questionnaire (OR, 2.6), being overweight (OR, 1.3) or neutered (OR, 3.6), previous surgery other than neutering (OR, 21.1), and the interaction between neuter status and previous surgery other than neutering (OR, 0.1) were associated with the odds of pancreatitis.

The breeds of the dogs within the study were not described, but there were comments in the discussion that there was no association between sporting breeds and miniature poodles [7].

The paper did discuss the limitations of the study using a control group with renal disease. It was not commented on what diet the control group of renal dogs consumed. It should be noted that renal diets have a higher fat content in comparison to life-stage diets. Animals suffering from renal compromise are often dysorexic; in some cases, this can lead to anorexia, so owners often feed high-fat treats and table scraps. This could therefore falsely decrease the measure of association between certain dietary factors and pancreatitis, hence making it more difficult to identify a significant relationship in the statistical analysis.

James et al. [20] studied various enzymes associated with pancreatic response to the fat content of different diets. Ten healthy staff-owned dogs were used for the study, and inclusion in the study required no history of any pancreatic or gastrointestinal disturbances. The results were analysed by use of a repeated-measures general ANOVA, with a significance set at a value of $p \leq 0.05$. Results of this study showed no significant effect of the content of fat or the presence or absence of supplemental pancreatic enzymes and medium-chained triglycerides (MCTs) on the degree of pancreatic stimulation (assessed by measurement of serum canine trypsin-like immunoreactivity (cTLI), canine pancreatic lipase immunoreactivity (cPLI) and gastrin concentrations) in healthy dogs. There were some differences in the diets, but not a significant difference ($p = 0.33$). In all the diets, the MCT content, not type, was investigated; differences in fat type would be of interest in their pancreatic response. Pancreatic response in unhealthy animals could have the potential to be different and would prove to be of interest to be investigated. These results were similar to those of Czako et al. [21] that found that only in severe (necrotising) pancreatitis cases that the fat content of the diet did play an important role. The study demonstrated that the high-cholesterol diet did not damage the exocrine pancreas and didn't alter the course of acute oedematous pancreatitis, but it did aggravate acute necrotising pancreatitis. In healthy rats in the Czako et al. [21] study, there was no change in outcomes when fed different diets.

There are large ethical implications to take into consideration when investigating any treatment intervention for a disease process that is potentially life-threatening and notoriously painful. The retrospective study of Watson et al. [19] and Lem et al. [7] looked at the clinical and dietary history, so there is no issue with a control pancreatitis group that didn't receive treatment. In the other studies that were investigated, James et al. [20] looked at healthy individuals, so there were no ethical issues with a control group not receiving pain medication or other treatments. Czako et al. [21] studied rats, rather than dogs; no details were given on the ethical element of any analgesics given to the rats suffering from pancreatitis, oedematous pancreatitis and the necrotising pancreatitis.

CONCLUSION

A causal relationship between the use of high-fat diets and pancreatitis in canines has not been confirmed by these clinical papers. Canines who develop hypertriglyceridaemia (whether primary or secondary) are at a potential risk of developing pancreatitis (acute or chronic), and therefore a diet with an appropriate fat level and an appropriate type of fat that doesn't induce hypertriglyceridaemia would be beneficial, according to anecdotal evidence [19]. Higher fat diets have been shown to increase the exocrine pancreatic secretions [1, 2] and to increase the severity of necrotising pancreatitis in rats [21].

The type of dietary fat may play a more important role than the overall fat content, but whether this is of benefit in the treatment of pancreatitis is not known. Although there is no evidence that restriction of dietary fat alters pancreatic stimulation, restriction of dietary fat in dogs that have a confirmed history of pancreatitis is an important recommendation. Further studies would be required to adequately investigate the feeding of low-fat diets (fat levels and fat types) to all dogs with pancreatitis.

RELEVANCE TO VETERINARY PRACTICE

There is no direct control group evidence. Studies support the use of low-fat diets for those dogs with pancreatitis (or predisposing factors for it). More clinical research is required to look at causation links and whether correlations are in fact causation. Anecdotal evidence by leading specialists in internal medicine and pancreatitis does support the use of these diets, including one of the papers examined. As pancreatitis can lead to extreme abdominal discomfort and, in severe forms, be fatal, the lack of supporting evidence-based studies shouldn't remove the weighting of anecdotal evidence. Unsupported recommendations often quote diets with less than 10% fat on a dry matter basis (less than 17% of calories from fat) to be low fat, while diets with 10–15% fat (17–23% of calories) are considered to contain a moderate amount of fat. Foods with more than 20% fat are considered high-fat. When giving nutritional advice to clients with dogs with pancreatitis, low-fat diets (<10% fat on a DMB) should be recommended. Some veterinary diets, designed for dogs with pancreatitis, can have levels as low as 4% DMB. Some clients will need guidance on what foods to use or avoid for their pet.

Key Points

- Knowledge of predisposing factors to pancreatitis can aid in preventing any bouts from being induced.
- Preventing, identifying and resolving hyperlipidaemia will reduce the risk of pancreatitis.
- In cases where predisposition exists (hyperlipidaemia, certain breeds and obesity), other causal factors (hypotensive events and high-lipid foods) should be avoided.

REFERENCES

1. Haig, T.H. (1970). Pancreatic digestive enzymes: influence of a diet that augments pancreatitis. *J. Surg. Res.* 10: 601–607.
2. Yago, M.D., Martinez-Victoria, E., and Huertas, R.J. (1997). Effects of the amount and type of dietary fat on exocrine pancreatic secretion in dogs after different periods of adaptation. *Arch. Physiol. Biochem.* 105: 78–85.

3. Watson, P. (2015). Pancreatitis in dogs and cats: definitions and pathophysiology. *J. Small Anim. Pract.* 56: 3–12.
4. Xenoulis, P.G. (2015). Diagnosis of pancreatitis in dogs and cats. *J. Small Anim. Pract.* 56: 13–26.
5. Watson, P.J., Roulois, A.J., and Scase, T. (2007). Prevalence and breed distribution of chronic pancreatitis at post-mortem examination in first-opinion dogs. *J. Small Anim. Pract.* 28: 609–618.
6. Watson, P.J. (2012). Chronic pancreatitis in dogs. *Top. Companion Anim. Med.* 27: 133–139.
7. Lem, K.Y., Fosgate, G.T., Norby, B. et al. (2008). Associations between dietary factors and pancreatitis in dogs. *J. Am. Vet. Med. Assoc.* 233: 1425–1431.
8. Hess, R.S., Kass, P., and Shofer, F.S. (1999). Evaluation of risk factors for fatal acute pancreatitis in dogs. *J. Am. Vet. Med. Assoc.* 214: 46–51.
9. Xenoulis, P.G. and Steiner, J.M. (2010). Lipid metabolism and hyperlipidemia in dogs. *Vet. J.* 183: 12–21.
10. Gaskill, C.L. and Cribb, A.E. (2000). Pancreatitis associated with potassium bromide/phenobarbital combination therapy in epileptic dogs. *Can. Vet. J.* 41: 555.
11. Moriello, K.A., Bowen, D., and Meyer, D.J. (1987). Acute pancreatitis in two dogs given azathioprine and prednisolone. *J. Am. Vet. Med. Assoc.* 191: 695–696.
12. German, A.J. (2011). Canine Obesity – weighing on the mind on the owner? *J. Small Anim. Pract.* 52: 619–620.
13. Kim, D.I., Kim, H., Son, P. et al. (2017). Serum 25-hydroxyvitamin D concentrations in dogs with suspected acute pancreatitis. *J. Vet. Med. Sci.* 79 (8): 1366–1373.
14. Frenkel, D. (2007). Why does hyperlipidemic cause pancreatitis? *The NYU Langone Online. J. Med.* `https://www.clinicalcorrelations.org/?p=478` (accessed 4 August 2026).
15. Mori, N., Lee, P., Muranaka, S. et al. (2009). Predisposition for primary hyperlipidemia in Miniature Schnauzers and Shetland sheepdogs as compared to other canine breeds. *Res. Vet. Sci.* 88: 394–399.
16. DeMarco, V., Noronha, K.S.M., Casado, T.C. et al. (2017). Therapy of canine hyperlipidemia with bezafibrate. *J. Vet. Intern. Med.* 31: 717–722.
17. Xenoulis, P.G. and Steiner, J.M. (2015). Canine hyperlipidaemia. *J. Small Anim. Pract.* 56: 595–605.
18. Tsuang, W., Navaneethan, U., Ruiz, L. et al. (2009). Hypertriglyceridemic pancreatitis: presentation and management. *Am. J. Gastroenterol.* 104: 984–991.
19. Watson, P.J., Archer, J., Roulois, A.J. et al. (2010). Observation study of 14 cases of chronic pancreatitis in dogs. *Vet. Rec.* 167: 968–976.
20. James, F.E., Mansfield, C.S., Steiner, J.M. et al. (2009). Pancreatic response in healthy dogs fed diets of various fat compositions. *Am. J. Vet. Res.* 70 (5): 614–618.
21. Czakó, L., Szabolcs, A., Vajda, A. et al. (2007). Hyperlipidemia induced by a cholesterol-rich diet aggravates necrotizing pancreatitis in rats. *Eur. J. Pharmacol.* 572: 74–81.

Hydration

Certain clinical diseases or disorders require increased quantities of water in the diet. Encouraging an animal to increase its water intake can be difficult, and several methods may be required to achieve sufficient amounts.

Some animals can be extremely fastidious in what, when, and where they eat or drink. To increase water consumption, the availability of water needs to be improved. This can be achieved by placing more water bowls around the cat's environment (both inside and outside the house), using different types of water. Tap water, which is chlorinated, smells even more so to a cat or a dog. Allowing the water to stand for a period can remove a large portion of the chlorine and make it more palatable to the cat. Cats, which live in a multi-cat household, can find eating and drinking alongside other cats very intimidating. Making food and water available in a place that the particular cat feels safe can benefit them.

The water content of the diet should also be increased; this can involve changing the pet over to a moist diet or adding water to a moist diet. Some animals do not tend to consume dry biscuits that have had water added to them. The volume of water that needs to be added to kibbles to make a difference to the daily water total intake is high. Moist diets are normally approximately 80% and dry diets 8%, a 10-fold difference. If the water level of the diet is less than 60%, cats need additional drinking water. A mature cat must consume 60 ml/kg/day of water to maintain its body functions without any problem.

NUTRIENT-ENRICHED WATER PRODUCTS

Nutrient-enriched water refers to water that has had nutrients, like essential minerals, vitamins or other beneficial substances, added to it. ProPlan HydraCare includes organic osmolytes, including amino acids from whey protein, which play a role in fluid balance and cell volume and are absorbed into the body after consumption. Rather than increasing the circulating volume, these osmolytes help to increase the fluid volume within the cells. In animals that have polyuria due to the inability to prevent dehydration (for example, cats with renal insufficiency), this can help to maintain hydration.

The acceptance of nutrient-enriched water resulted in increased total water intake, and this was sustained over time [1, 2]. Urine volume was also increased and remained more dilute. The addition of the water supplement increased total water intake to 35–55 ml/kg bodyweight – on average 27% more than when dry food and water alone were offered [2]. This compares to a total water intake of 20–30 ml/kg bodyweight when dry food is fed, or 35 ml/kg bodyweight when wet food is fed [2]. There was a 48% increase in total daily urine volume compared to cats drinking tap water [1, 2].

WATER FOUNTAINS AND BOWLS

The importance of a complete nutritional history (that includes hydration elements) is important. Understanding how best the pet prefers to drink (running water, bowls, etc.) will help give recommendations for how we can increase water consumption. Cats that prefer running water will use water fountains; not all cats will [3]. A study looking at water fountains and water consumption showed that cats that like water fountains will drink more water. If the cat had no history or had shown no interest in drinking running water, it showed no interest in using a water fountain [3]. Other research has shown similar outcomes, looking at differences between bowl shape, size and movement of water [4, 5]. Cats have preferences, but it won't produce a statistically significant increase in water consumption [4, 5].

WATER VISCOSITY

The viscosity (thickness) of the water does help to increase the amount that is consumed [6]. Lapping occurs by fluid adhesion to the dorsal part of the tongue's tip and by lifting a liquid column through the tongue's upward motion before jaw closure. Water with a higher viscosity enables more to be lifted into the mouth.

WATER TEMPERATURE

Temperature is considered to be very important for the taste perception of animals. The preference for the water temperature varies among the animal species. Studies have shown in cats that adding a couple of ice cubes to the water bowl will increase water consumption [7], though conflicting studies have shown that warm water increases consumption [8]. The clinical history of the animal can also affect the preference for cold or warm water. Cold water can help soothe pain/inflammation in the mouth.

The use of flavoured waters can tempt some animals, but be careful of brands that are high in sugar. Ice cubes can also be used and are especially useful in hot temperatures. Stocks can be high in different types of salts, not just sodium. Water from tins of tuna is commonly offered to pets. Tuna brine should be avoided due to the high salt content; however, even tuna in spring water should also be avoided, as tuna can contain high levels of heavy metals.

Commercially produced broths can have great effects in increasing water consumption and are being produced with restricted levels of phosphates (ideal for renal patients) and sodium. Some even contain hydrolysed proteins.

Increasing water consumption is a very individualised process. The species, age, clinical history and individual preferences play a large role in increasing consumption. Taking the nutritional history (including hydration elements) is vital to find out these preferences.

REFERENCES

1. Zanghi, B.M., Wils-Plotz, E., DeGeer, S., and Gardner, C.L. (2018). Effects of a nutrient-enriched water with and without poultry flavoring on water intake, urine specific gravity, and urine output in healthy domestic cats fed a dry kibble diet. *Am. J. Vet. Res.* 79 (11): 1150–1159.
2. Zanghi, B.M., Gerheart, L., and Gardner, C.L. (2018). Effects of a nutrient-enriched water on water intake and indices of hydration in healthy domestic cats fed a dry kibble diet. *Am. J. Vet. Res.* 79 (7): 733–744.
3. Christopher, P. and Jacqui, N. (2010). Comparison of feline water consumption between still and flowing water sources: a pilot study. *J. Vet. Behav.* 5 (3): 130–133.
4. Robbins, M.T., Cline, M.G., Bartges, J.W. et al. (2018). Quantified water intake in laboratory cats from still, free-falling and circulating water bowls, and its effects on selected urinary parameters. *J. Feline Med. Surg.* 21 (8): 682–690. https://doi.org/10.1177/1098612X18803753.
5. Grant, D.C. (2010). Effect of water source on intake and urine concentration in healthy cats. *J. Feline Med. Surg.* 12 (6): 431–434. https://doi.org/10.1016/j.jfms.2009.10.008.
6. Hall, J.A., Vanchina, M.A., Ogleby, B., and Jewell, D.E. (2021). Increased water viscosity enhances water intake and reduces risk of calcium oxalate stone formation in cats. *Animals* 11 (7): 2110. https://doi.org/10.3390/ani11072110.
7. Tatlıağız, Z. and Akyazı, İ. (2023). Investigation of the effect of water temperature on water consumption of cats. *J. Istanbul Vet. Sci.* 7 (1): 50–54. https://doi.org/10.30704/http-www-jivs-net.1278513.
8. Eyre, R., Trehiou, M., Marshall, E. et al. (2022). Aging cats prefer warm food. *J. Vet. Behav.* 47: 86–92.

Abbreviations

AAFCO	Association of American Feed Control Officials
ACE	angiotensin-converting enzyme
AFR	adverse food reaction
ATP	adenosine triphosphate
BCS	body condition score
BER	basal energy requirements
BUN	blood urea nitrogen
BV	biological value
BWT	body weight
CHF	chronic heart failure
CRT	capillary refill time
DCM	dilated cardiomyopathy
DE	digestible energy
DER	daily energy requirements
DHA	docosahexaenoic acid
DNA	deoxyribonucleic acid
ECG	electrocardiogram
EFA	essential fatty acid
EPA	eicosapentaenoic acid
EPI	exocrine pancreatic insufficiency
FLUTD	Feline lower urinary tract disorder/disease
GE	gross energy
HE	hepatic encephalopathy
IBD	inflammatory bowel disease
IBS	Irritable Bowel Syndrome
Ig	immunoglobulin
IRIS	International Renal Interest Society
MCS	muscle condition score
MCT	medium-chained triglyceride
ME	metabolisable energy
OA	osteoarthritis
PEG	percutaneous endoscopic gastrostomy
PPH	parts per hundred
PPM	parts per million
PPS	portal systemic shunt
PTH	parathyroid hormone
QOL	quality of life
RCVS	Royal College of Veterinary Surgeons
RER	resting energy requirements
ROS	reactive oxygen species
RVN	Registered Veterinary Nurse (UK)

SCFA	short-chain fatty acid
SDMA	symmetric dimethylarginine
SGLT2	sodium-glucose cotransporter-2
SQP	suitably qualified person
SVN	student veterinary nurse
TCA	tricarboxylic acid
VFA	volatile fatty acid
VN	veterinary nurse
VS	veterinary surgeon
WSAVA	World Small Animal Veterinary Association

Glossary

Absorption: The uptake of an ingested substance from the gastrointestinal tract into the villi of the tract.

Acceptability: A measure of whether a recommendation/product/diet/idea meets the requirements of the individual and is accepted.

Ad Lib: Ad libitum, unrestricted or freely available, quantity and time are not restricted.

Aerophagia: The habit of swallowing air whilst eating.

An-: Prefix meaning none, absence or stopped.

Anorexia: The complete lack or loss of appetite.

Anthropomorphic: Attributing human-based perceptions to the pet's needs or preferences.

Anuria: No production or excretion of urine.

Ascites: The abnormal accumulation of serous fluid in the abdominal cavity.

Atopy: Genetic tendency to develop allergic reactions, often related to pruritus.

Availability (bioavailability): The degree to which a drug or nutrient becomes available to the target tissue after administration or consumption.

Azotaemia: Presence of excess nitrogen-containing compounds in the blood.

Bacterial translocation: Bacteria move from one place (the gut lumen) into another (the bloodstream) because of mucosal breakdown.

Biome: A large naturally occurring community of flora and fauna occupying a specific area, for example, gastrointestinal tract, skin or ear.

Bolus: An amount given in one set volume – this can relate to medications, fluids and food.

Borborygmus: Noises from the abdomen associated with gas or fluids passing through the intestinal tract.

Brachycephalic: Describes the conformation of the head – being shorter. Can relate to dogs, cats and rabbits.

Cachexia: A profound state of general ill health and starvation, characterised by severe body wasting.

Caecum: The proximal part of the large intestine.

Calculus: Calcified plaque on the tooth surface.

Cholangiohepatitis: Inflammation of the biliary ducts and liver.

Colitis: Inflammation of the colon.

Colon: The section of the large intestine extending from the caecum to the rectum. Can be divided into the ascending, transverse and descending sections.

Colonocytes: Cells lining the colon.

Colostrum: The 'first milk' produced after parturition that contains maternal antibodies.

Constipation: Hard, dry faeces passed infrequently and with difficulty.

Coprophagy: Habit of eating faeces.

Diuresis: Increased removal/excretion of fluid.

Duodenum: The proximal part of the small intestine

Dys-: Prefix meaning difficult,

Dystocia: Difficulty in giving birth.

Eclampsia: A condition where convulsions occur during pregnancy in hypertensive patients.

Eicosanoid: A compound derived from arachidonic acid, for example, prostaglandin

Electrolyte: A substance that when mixed in water dissociates into charged ions.

Encephalopathy: Any degenerative disease of the brain.

Endocrine: Relating to or denoting glands which secrete hormones or other products directly into the blood.

Energy density: The concentration of energy in a particular food or nutrient.

Enteral: Referring to the upper alimentary tract.

Enteritis: Inflammation of the small intestine.

Exocrine: Relating to or denoting glands which secrete their products through ducts opening onto an epithelium rather than directly into the blood.

Fermentation: The digestion of nutrients by anaerobic microorganisms.

Gastrocolic reflex: Involves increased motility of the colon in response to stretch in the stomach and byproducts of digestion in the small intestine. Thus, this reflex is responsible for the urge to defecate following a meal.

Gluten: A protein found in all cereals except rice

Hormone: A protein messenger within the body that can be endocrine or exocrine in origin, will have either a positive or negative feedback mechanism.

Hyper-: Prefix meaning above, an increase or excessive

Hypo-: Prefix meaning below, a decrease or deficiency.

Icterus: Jaundice, the yellowing of mucus membranes or skin.

Ileum: The distal portion of the small intestine.

Immunocompetence: The ability to develop an immune response after exposure to an antigen.

Integument: The skin and hair

Jejunum: Portion of the small intestine from the duodenum to the ileum.

Ketone: A metabolic product derived from the breakdown of fatty acids.

Ketotic: Accumulation of ketones in the bloodstream.

Lactulose: A disaccharide (sugar) of galactose and fructose. It cannot be hydrolysed (broken down) by mammalian enzymes but can be fermented in the colon by the biome.

Lipid: Group of compounds that include oils, fats and waxes.

Lumen: A cavity or channel.

Megacolon: Lack of muscle tone and dilation of the colon.

Megaoesophagus: Lack of muscle tone and dilation of the oesophagus.

Melaena: The presence of digested blood in the faeces, resulting in black tarry stools.

Metabolism: The chemical processes that occur within a living organism to maintain life

Microbiota: The microorganisms of a particular site.

Mobility: The ability to move.

Morphometry: The measurement of the structures and parts of organisms.

Nares: Singular naris, opening of the nasal cavity.

Neoplasm: Any new or abnormal growth.

Nephron: The structural and functional unit within the kidney.

Nutraceutical: A supplement, derived from nutrients, that has therapeutic benefits.

Obligate: has to be

Oedema: An abnormal accumulation of fluid in the cavities and intercellular spaces of the body.

Oesophagitis: Inflammation of the oesophagus.

Oliguria: Abnormally low levels of urine being produced.

Osteoclasts: Cells that remove bone.

Otitis: Inflammation of the ear. Can be split into externa (outer) or media (middle).

Palatability: A measure of how much something is liked or not, often related to food.

Pheromones: Hormone-like substances secreted by an individual, affecting the behaviours of others within the same species.

Pica: Craving or eating unusual substances.

Poly-: Prefix meaning more or many.

Polydipsia: Excessive thirst

Polyuria: Increases the production and excretion of urine.

Postbiotic: A preparation of nonliving microorganisms or their components that may have health benefits.

Postprandial: After eating

Prebiotic: A nondigestible food ingredient that promotes the growth of beneficial microorganisms in the intestines.

Probiotic: Live microorganisms promoted with claims that they provide health benefits when consumed, generally by improving or restoring the gut microbiota.

Pruritic: Itchy

Sarcopenia: Muscle wastage

Satiety: Having fulfilled all desires to eat and drink.

Steatorrhoea: The presence of fats in the faeces.

Struvite: A type of crystal or urolith that forms in the bladder, magnesium-ammonium-phosphate hexahydrate or triple phosphate.

Supplement: An addition to the basic food.

Synbiotic: A combination of probiotics, prebiotics and/or postbiotics that can improve the health of the gut and body.

Tenesmus: The act of straining to pass urine or faeces.

Uraemia: An excess of urea, creatinine and other nitrogenous waste products in the blood; also termed azotaemia.

Urea: The main nitrogenous end product of protein metabolism, formed in the liver from amino acids and ammonia compounds.

Urethritis: Inflammation of the urethra.

Urolith: A calculus (stone) in the urine or urinary tract.

Urolithiasis: The formation of calculi in the urinary tract.

Index

Note: Page numbers with f refer to figures and t refer to tables.